Documentation
SKILLS

For
Quality Patient Care

DOCUMENTATION
SKILLS

For
Quality Patient Care

By
Fay Yocum, R.N.

Awareness Productions
Tipp City, Ohio

Published by: **Awareness Productions**
P.O. Box 85
Tipp City, Ohio 45371-0085

Printed by: **Wickersham Printing Co., Inc.**

Editor: **Esther Silverman**

Legal Consultant: **Sue Dill Calloway, R.N., J.D.**

Cover Design: **Steve Karmele**

Disclaimer

This book discusses the provision of quality patient care through nursing documentation. In the course of this discussion, examples of treatment and medications are given. These examples are not intended in any way to provide recommendations or medical advice regarding treatment or pharmacology for any condition. Any practice or technique described in this book should be applied by the reader in accordance with the professional standards of care appropriate in the unique circumstances of the situation. The author, editors, and publisher are not responsible for errors or omissions or for consequences from application of the book, and make no warranty expressed or implied regarding the contents of this book.

Library of Congress Catalog Card Number: 93-79567
ISBN 0-9637649-7-7: $18.95 Softcover

10 9 8 7 6 5 4 3 2 1

Dedication

This book is dedicated to the memory of my mother, Isabell Ellen Snyder Yocum, who encouraged me to meet all challenges head on and to learn from them. To say the least, this book has been a challenge and I have learned a lot.

I hope you will use this book to meet the challenges you face in your nursing career. In this way I can share a little of my mother's love and encouragement with you.

Table of Contents

Example List of
Nursing Notes

Other examples are located in the exercises and test.

Foreword

Charting is a means of documenting the nursing care rendered. Among the many reasons for creating and maintaining good medical records are the following:

1. To serve as a basis for planning the patient's care and for continuity in evaluating the patient's condition and treatment.
2. To furnish evidence of the course of the patient's medical evaluation, treatment, and change in condition.
3. To provide documentation to obtain reimbursement.
4. To document communication among the practitioners responsible for the patient's care.
5. To provide data for use in education, research, peer review studies, quality improvement, and assessment.
6. To create a legal record for the patient.

While all of these reasons are important, the last one is often overlooked in many nursing curriculum programs. Good documentation is one of the most important strategies for keeping the nurse out of the courtroom. The patient's medical record is a legal record that can be introduced into the courtroom as evidence. Good concise charting can be the nurse's best defense in a malpractice suit. The medical record's content can determine the outcome of the case if a lawsuit is filed.

One court warned nurses that the availability and accuracy of the medical records is not a mere technicality, but a legal requirement. *Valcin v. Public Health Trust of Dade County*, 3rd District, Case No. 91-2131 (Fla. 1984).

Many nurses have heard the phrase "If it wasn't documented, it wasn't done." In the case of *Stack v. Wapner*, the court held that where there were no notations by the physician of a woman in labor, the jury could conclude that no monitoring occurred. 368 A. 2d 292 (Pa. 1976). The courts have also held that lack of documentation implies lack of care. *Wagner v. Kaiser Foundation Hospital*, 589 P. 2d 1106 (Or. 1979). Many cases have been decided on the adequacy of the nurse's charting. *Mastonka v. Herman*, 414 A. 2d 135 (N.J. Super. Ct. 1980). These cases illustrate the legal importance of good documentation.

Many students are not aware that good documentation can directly prevent the filing of a lawsuit. Most states now provide the patient with access to a copy of their medical records. A disgruntled or angry patient may seek the services of an attorney. The attorney may have the patient sign a medical records release form. This form is sent to the hospital's medical records department. A copy of the records is generally sent to the patient's attorney. The attorney then will mail the hospital records to a reviewing expert who is a nurse, physician, or other appropriate health care practitioner. Most often, the decision made to sue is based on the simple review of the medical records by the plaintiff's. That is why the importance of documentation should never by underestimated.

This book contains many excellent tips on documentation, as well as a discussion of many of the national standards that have an impact on documentation. Additionally, the book addresses many practical pointers on documentation that might take years of practical experience to acquire.

SUE DILL CALLOWAY, RN, JD

Acknowledgment

I wish to thank the following people and organizations:

Sharon Boatwright the Director of Nurses at Wayne Memorial Hospital, Jesup, Georgia who issued me "a challenge". The nurses at Wayne Memorial Hospital who then rose to the greater challenge.

Betty Morton and Geneva Bible who encouraged, read, reread, suggested, and encouraged some more. They have perfected the swift kick to a fine art of motivation and achievement. Barbara Fisher, Karen Sorrow, and Charlene Hand who helped me get started.

The librarians at Troy and Tipp City, Ohio Public Libraries, Wright Patterson Air Force Base Medical Library, Fordham Health Sciences Library Wright State University, and Health Sciences Library of Department of Veteran Affairs Medical Center at Dayton, Ohio, for their ability to find whatever information, I needed.

My editor who took a manuscript from a dyslexic writer and turned it into a readable book. I'm just sorry she could not turn it into a comedy! Sue Dill Calloway who did the legal review. Steve Karmele who designed the cover and guided the book layout. The Aldus Technical Support staff, Page Maker 5.0, who were always available, knowledgeable, helpful, and friendly.

Other reviewers including Alice Cox, Cathy Foster, John Jezierski, Debbie McMillan, Susan Lampe, Cheryl Udensi, and Janet Weber.

Don Lee and his staff on 2 North and others at The 645th Medical Group, Wright Patterson Air Force Base, for listening to me talk about the book and for their continuing encouragement.

What I owe my family is far too much to list here. Suffice it to say that without them this book would probably never have happened, especially not in twelve months from start to finish.

Others have helped along the way, and I want them to know their help was greatly appreciated.

Thank you to one and all!

Introduction

Documentation and documentation skills are as essential for quality nursing care as providing emotional support, teaching a patient self-care, or giving an injection. Documentation should not be regarded as a nuisance task to be completed as quickly as possible at the end of a long day. Rather, it should be viewed as providing important patient information that is vital for quality patient care, your legal self-protection, and your agency's self-interests.

This manual is written for students and professional nurses who want to develop or strengthen existing documentation skills. The goal of the manual is to help the learner write clear, complete, and concise nurses' notes that demonstrate the discharging of the nurse's professional responsibilities to the patient and to the institution.

Nurses and nursing have faced many changes and have grown in many ways in the last decades. Some of these changes that have affected documentation are:

1. Patients are no longer passive; they demand to know what is being done to or for them.

Documentation and documentation skills are as essential for quality nursing care as providing emotional support, teaching a patient self-care, or giving an injection.

1

2. Hospitals are being run more like businesses than charity institutions that dispense care based on humanitarian needs only.
3. Patients admitted to health care facilities are sicker than ever before and have shorter hospital stays.
4. More patients are receiving technical care formerly provided in hospitals at home or in nursing homes.
5. Large settlements and verdicts are often made in the patient's favor.
6. Technology is constantly changing, challenging a nurse's ability to stay current.
7. Health care costs are spiraling out of control; and government, industry, and individuals are struggling to make health care affordable and available.

Each of these changes have in one way or another affected nursing documentation and the way in which nurses perform their job. In spite of these changes, the nurse and nursing services must meet established standards of care.

In this changing world of medicine and nursing, nurses are assuming many new responsibilities in addition to their old ones. Documentation is only one of many nursing responsibilities and has always been difficult. Trouble arises in knowing when to document, what to document, and how to word what you want to say. There never seems to be enough time to write as much as you need or want. In addition, a nurse who is responsible for as many as 20 patients will often be interrupted, making it difficult to complete documentation properly or even to maintain a train of thought. Finally, the same piece of information may need to be documented more than once. Despite these problems, important information must be documented to meet patient needs, your needs, and those of your employer.

Nurses have often been heard complaining, *"Why do I have to document when no one ever reads what I write."* Or, *"I could go home now if I didn't have to chart."* We need to remember though that as nurses we have a unique relationship with the patient. We spend the most time with each patient and have the greatest opportunity to gather and disseminate information vital to his/her well-being. We must regard documentation as a method to provide quality patient care, not as a nuisance task.

Strong professional documentation is the responsibility not only of the nurse, but also of Nursing Administration and Nursing Education. The nurse must write clear concise accurate nursing notes at the appropriate time. (S)he must meet the standards of documentation as set by the hospital, Nurse Practice Act, professional organizations, and accrediting bodies. Finally, the nurse must be open to new learning experiences and changes in the profession.

Nursing Administration must create and maintain a viable system that fosters expedient and complete documentation. Forms must be available that are complete, easy to use, concise, and consistent. Double documentation and other time-consuming practices must be identified and corrected. The time allocated for documentation must be determined realistically when figuring staffing and acuity levels so that the nurse has time to document thoroughly.

Basic nursing education programs must provide the new nurse with the tools and skills to document in their new profession. Education must also help keep current practitioners up to date and refine skills as the requirements for documentation change. Education should also provide a bridge between the staff nurses and Nursing Administration to help identify and solve problems with current documentation practices.

Nursing Administration, Education, and staff nurses must generate an attitude toward documentation that goes beyond

Your first responsibility when documenting is to include information vital to providing your patient the best care possible in the shortest time and at the least expense.

the notion that its only purpose is to provide legal protection. Strong documentation should be thought of as a key element in providing quality patient care.

This manual is organized into nine chapters. Information is arranged so that you can quickly find the chapter containing the information you are seeking.

When documenting patient care, you must be sure to legally protect yourself and your employer. There is no way around this fact. But remember, you became a nurse to help people. Your first responsibility when documenting is to include information vital to providing your patient the best care possible in the shortest time and at the least expense. You need to communicate with other health care team members in a clear, concise manner to ensure a proper plan of care both during and after your direct care involvement.

You need to communicate with other health care team members in a clear, concise manner to ensure a proper plan of care both during and after your direct care involvement.

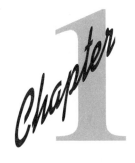

Chapter 1

Meeting Patient and Professional Needs and Regulations

Objectives

The learner will be able to:
1. Explain the American Nurses' Association 1980 definition of nursing.
2. Identify whose needs are met through appropriate nursing documentation.
3. List reasons for nursing documentation.
4. Discuss how regulations and regulatory bodies relate to nursing documentation.

Quality care is not only the gentle hand on a shoulder, a sterile dressing change, or a successful code; it is also the clear, concise, and complete documentation of the facts.

Documentation, one of the most important responsibilities in nursing, is necessary to meet patient needs, your needs, and the needs of the agency or institution. It is one way to demonstrate professional competency and the ability to discharge your responsibilities to the patient and employer. Clear, concise nursing documentation of patient care communicates who the patient is, what nursing care was provided, and the patient's response to that care. Always remember that nursing documentation is a component of patient care. Quality care is not only the gentle hand on a shoulder, a sterile dressing change, or a successful code; it is also the clear, concise, and complete documentation of the facts.

5

Nursing diagnoses change as the patient's condition improves or deteriorates.

The definition of nursing, its standards, and legal requirements differentiate nurses from doctors. These criteria guide the practice of nursing and tell the consumer what can be expected from a nurse or nursing service. As a student of nursing, you should learn about the definition, standards, and legal requirements to better understand why you require certain learning experiences and have certain responsibilities. To understand why Nursing Administration and Education make specific decisions and set certain requirements, you need to realize that in most cases, Nursing Administration and Education are responding to changes in the field of nursing, consumer expectations, and governing policies.

Nursing as a profession is always growing and changing. A 1936 graduate of a nursing program reports she was not taught how to take blood pressure readings during her training. She did not learn to perform this task until the early 1940s. Today nurses with specialized education deliver babies, administer anesthesia, and provide health consulting to mention only a few advanced nursing skills. These changes have been reflected in the area of nursing documentation. Nurses making nursing diagnoses must state exactly what they observe and plan for patient care.

Nursing has been defined by the American Nurses' Association in its 1980 *Nursing: A Social Policy Statement:* **"...the diagnosis and treatment of human responses to actual or potential health problems."**[1] This definition is important to understand because it clarifies the actions that are performed for the patient, whether the patient is an individual, group, or society. Doctors treat a pathologic condition such as pneumonia. Nurses diagnose and treat the patient's response to the pneumonia—that is, the impaired gas exchange, pain, or high risk for altered body temperature—but not the pneumonia itself. A doctor's diagnosis, once made, usually stays the same. Nursing diagnoses change as the patient's condition improves or deteriorates. The initial focus may be the impaired gas exchange, pain, and fever; but as the patient improves, the focus may transfer to teaching.

The ANA's definition is the nursing profession's definition of nursing. Each state has its own legal definition of nursing, which is set forth in the state's Nurse Practice Act. (See the section State Board of Nursing later in this chapter.)

Documentation is defined by *Webster's Third New International Dictionary* as: "The use of historical documents especially in the writing of history or of works relying on the authenticity of historical information."[2] As a nurse, you are required by various regulations and standards to document information about the patient. The information gathered is documented as a "history" of events, which will be reviewed by other nurses, doctors, social workers, and utilization review personnel, among others, to plan future actions and evaluate care rendered. These records are also used in research, education, continuous quality improvement, and financial reimbursement. Medical records help the patient now and in the future. Examination of past and current patient records can help the nurse "make a difference" in a patient's progress. You never know when one reported fact will provide information to confirm a diagnosis or a better understanding of the patient's problem.

The medical record includes all pieces of information compiled about a particular patient. The types of records kept vary depending on the clinical setting. A hospital record includes, but is not limited to, nurse's progress notes, nursing flow sheets, doctor's orders, doctor's progress notes, laboratory results, x-ray study reports, and notes by other health team members. A record in the doctor's office may consist of several pages of doctor's notes and laboratory reports. A hospital record can quickly become a large volume, depending on the reason for hospitalization and length of stay. Those earlier medical records are often requested on sequence admissions to establish continuity of care and to assess changes in a patient's condition.

Remember: What you document today may, in later years, influence the care given. On many occasions, I have reviewed records to assess the changes in a patient's condition. Documentation is not a last-minute nuisance task, but a way of providing high-quality patient care.

Meeting the Needs
The Patient

The primary reason for documentation must always be to provide high-quality patient care. The more thorough the documentation, the better the plan of care that the health care team can develop and implement. Proper documentation will enhance communication between nursing and others reading the notes by providing a complete picture of the patient. The note should be able to support your evaluations with enough information to help others understand exactly what you have observed.

Documentation should reflect patient treatment and care. In addition, notes should contain the following:

- Information related to patient teaching
- Patient's own words about his/her condition
- What your senses (hearing, sight, smell, taste, and touch) tell you
- The patient's response to the nursing treatment and care

It is important to document responses to treatment and care to evaluate the effectiveness of the plan of care. If a treatment is ineffective, an alternative treatment plan must be implemented.

Medical and nursing care in the hospital are provided on a 24 hour basis, and team members are rarely together at the same time. The medical record is the tool by which valuable information is communicated between team members. Because each team member approaches the patient from a different perspective and with different skills, each may

> **Documentation is not a last-minute nuisance task, but a way of providing high-quality patient care.**

REASONS FOR DOCUMENTATION

Provide quality care
Communicate between
  health team members
Describe care
  provided
Describe response to care
Evaluate care provided
Provide legal evidence
Provide data for
  research
Use in education
Use in Continuous
  Quality
  Improvement
Provide proof for
  reimbursement
Validate Diagnostic
  Related Group
  assignment
Prove medical necessity
  for admission and
  treatment
Identify patient's health
  status and changes
  therein
Document safety
  measures
Provide proof of meeting
  individual and institu-
  tional responsibilities

gather different information that you may have been unable to obtain. Documented information allows team members to assess changes, prove diagnoses, identify new needs, meet the patients' varied needs, and have a better understanding of the patient. Consider the following example.

On your first night back after vacation, Mr. Jones appears to be having so much trouble breathing that you are concerned, even though he says he is okay. You complete your initial assessment. You now need to know whether this observation indicates a change in the patient's condition. After reviewing Mr. Jones' chart you find that his condition is actually improved. The only way to find out that information and validate his input is by reviewing the documentation. Most nurses can recall a case when documentation was insufficient to make that assessment. This lack of documentation is not only extremely frustrating, it is potentially hazardous to the patient.

It is our responsibility as nurses to ensure that we have documented appropriately. Information that is properly documented in the record is a valuable resource for all team members in planning and providing patient care. The more information available, the better the plan of care, both during and after hospitalization. The following example illustrates how a nurse's failure to document caused a problem for the patient during discharge.

An elderly Native American was admitted with a fractured hip. During the admission process the database was not completed and that fact was not communicated. The patient was being discharged using a walker. It was learned on discharge that she lived in a traditional hogan (house) with no electricity, no flooring, or inside bathroom. She had to go outside over uneven terrain to go to the bathroom. Because the patient's home environment was not documented, the discharge had to be slightly delayed until appropriate help was arranged so that she could safely navigate the uneven terrain. (It should be noted that this example was a case of whole system failure, because the patient's living arrangements should have been explored by all departments working with her.)

All patients undergo a nursing admission assessment, usually within 24 hours after admission. If you cannot complete the assessment within the hospital's guidelines, the incomplete assessment must be noted and addressed by someone else. You responsibility is to make sure that the assessment is completed by proper communication.

Proper documentation is important to the patient legally. At times, patients have used their medical record to prove legal issues that have nothing to do with the care they received in the hospital. The medical record has been used to prove abuse, obtain custody of minors, prove workers' compensation claims, and support personal injury lawsuits after an accident.[3] The patient can also use the medical record to prove malpractice cases against the health care team.

A patient will file a lawsuit when (s)he has experienced a physical or an emotional injury. You can win or lose the case based on professionalism evidenced through your documentation.

Protecting Yourself

You must document adequately to protect yourself legally. Many nurses have given the proper care or responded to situations appropriately, but because they failed to document the care completely, they have lost a lawsuit.

The importance of the medical record cannot be overemphasized. It proves the nature and quality of care provided. The basic premise in a court of law is, "If it is not documented it was not done." Recently, a few cases have been won even though documentation was poor because other records provided proof of care.[4] Nevertheless, you should always document, so that you clearly describe what happened during your care of the patient.

The most important reason to document is to discharge your professional responsibilities to the patient by communicating completely with other care givers. A patient will file a lawsuit when (s)he has experienced a physical or an emotional injury. You can win or lose the case based on professionalism evidenced through your documentation. The information in the health record is regarded as proof of occurrence. Documentation that fails to show evidence that you discharged your professional responsibilities appropriately is no better than no documentation at all. At the very least, the lack of proper documentation places the nurse's credibility in jeopardy.

It is a good idea to acquire one of the many books about nursing and the law for your personal professional library. Review these books to obtain a better understanding of how nurses have won or lost lawsuits through their documentation. You can help protect yourself by learning from someone else's mistakes.

Agency or Institution

Proper documentation allows the institution to prove that it is meeting its obligations to the patient, society, patient's family, and health care professions. The agency or institution has obligations to provide safe, competent, quality, and cost-effective care. They must provide care that improves the patient's health status, maintains health, or allows the patient to die with dignity.

Third-party payers review records to ensure that the patient is billed for services. Not only must the proper billing procedures be followed, but the use of an item must be documented before the insurance company will pay. If large quantities of supplies are used, documentation must justify their use. Third-party payers will examine your nurses notes to be sure that the hospitalization or specific procedure was medically indicated. At one time, it was not unusual for a family caring for an elderly relative to hospitalize that relative while they went away on vacation. Although these persons did not require hospitalization, doctors would write orders and the patient was cared for. Under the current rules, there must be medical justification for an admission before an insurance company will pay for the hospitalization. The insurance companies will look at the nursing notes to help prove or disprove medical justification. If your notes denote custodial care only, the reimbursement may be denied.

Medical records are used for research, education, and continuous quality improvement programs and to improve skills, knowledge, and practice within the hospital and the health care profession.

Continuous quality improvement is vital to the survival of all businesses whether private, governmental, or health care related. An organization reviews records to determine whether it is meeting its own goals. Investigators review current practices in an attempt to make the business more efficient and cost-effective. To provide an affordable health care system we must constantly assess the way we do our job, the cost of doing business, and the cost to patients. Always try to work and use equipment as if you were paying for it.

Medicare instituted a program to determine how much they would pay for various services Medicare recipients received, which is called Diagnostic Related Groups (DRG). This system of classification groups related medical diagnosis into categories based on the amount of resources used for the patient with a particular diagnosis. Then payment was set for that group. If the cost exceeds the allowed amount, the hospital absorbs the cost. If it costs the hospital less to treat the patient, the hospital keeps the additional money. Your records will help the hospital verify the DRG category and aid in reimbursement from the government. The hospital categorizes the patient's diagnosis as indicated by the doctor. If government reviewers do not validate the doctor's diagnosis, they may move the patient to a different category, which could mean lose of reimbursement to the hospital and fewer hospital days for the patient. For example, the original diagnosis may allow seven days of hospitalization at a cost of $4,000. The new category may allow only five days of hospitalization at $3,000. Obviously, it is important for the hospital to be able to prove the original diagnosis. This proof is provided by appropriate documentation. You must remember that every dollar denied prevents the institution from buying necessary equipment, upgrading equipment, or enhancing your benefit package.

Medical records provide legal protection for the institution and the nurse. An inadequate record can put the institution in jeopardy of not being able to prove that appropriate care was given.

Reality Check

You will hear many comments in the clinical area about the need to chart to protect yourself legally. I challenge you to remember that strong documentation leads to quality patient care. Your first and foremost reason to document is to discharge your professional responsibilities to your patient by communicating completely with other care givers. Documentation is not a nuisance task to complete before going home. Rather, it is as important as giving medications and treatments and talking with the patient and family. Certainly, the legal ramifications of improper charting practices must be considered, but your concern should be quality care.

Regulators and Regulations

Every profession is supported by many organizations or agencies that set standards, rules, regulations, or laws governing its practice. The profession of nursing is regulated or supervised by the American Nurses' Association (ANA), state boards of nursing, Joint Commission on Accreditation of Healthcare Organizations (JCAHO), state and federal governments, special practice groups, and individual agencies or institutions. Failure to meet the standards of these groups have resulted in the loss of lawsuits and loss of JCAHO accreditation. An agency may discharge a health care professional who does not meet those standards, especially if that professional fails to improve after proper education and supervision.

American Nurses' Association

One of the responsibilities of the ANA, the professional nurses' organization, is the establishment of practice standards to protect the patient through the provision of high-quality nursing care. ANA standards are used to measure

Figure 1-1: STANDARDS OF CARE

Standard I. Assessment

THE NURSE COLLECTS CLIENT HEALTH DATA

  Measurement Criteria

   1. The priority of data collection is determined by the client's immediate condition or needs.

   2. Pertinent data are collected using appropriate assessment techniques.

   3. Data collection involves the client, significant others, and health care providers when appropriate.

   4. The data collection process is systematic and ongoing.

   5. *Relevant data are documented in a retrievable form.*

Standard II. Diagnosis

THE NURSE ANALYZES THE ASSESSMENT DATA IN DE-TERMINING DIAGNOSIS.

  Measurement Criteria

   1. Diagnoses are derived from the assessment data.

   2. Diagnoses are validated with the client, significant others, and health care providers, when possible.

   3. *Diagnoses are documented in a manner that facilitates the determination of expected outcomes and plan of care.*

Standard III. Outcome Identification

THE NURSE IDENTIFIES EXPECTED OUTCOMES INDIVIDUAL-IZED TO THE CLIENT.

  Measurement Criteria

   1. Outcomes are derived from the diagnosis.

   2. *Outcomes are documented as measurable goals.*

   3. Outcomes are mutually formulated with the client and health care providers, when possible.

   4. Outcomes are realistic in relation to the client's present and potential capabilities.

   5. Outcomes are attainable in relation to resources available to the client.

   6. Outcomes include a time estimate for attainment.

   7. Outcomes provide direction for continuity of care.

Standard IV. Planning

THE NURSE DEVELOPS A PLAN OF CARE THAT PRESCRIBES INTERVENTIONS TO ATTAIN EXPECTED OUTCOMES.

  Measurement Criteria

   1. The plan is individualized to the client's condition or needs.

   2. The plan is developed with the client, significant others, and health care providers, when appropriate.

Continued on the next page

the competence of the individual or organization to deliver quality nursing care. The nursing process is the foundation of the ANA's Standards of Care, addressing assessment, analysis (diagnosis), outcome identification, planning, implementation, and evaluation. Each standard has a title, definition, and measurement criteria. The measurement criteria describe the way in which the practitioner's or agency's competency is evaluated.

Within each of the six Standards of Care are measurement criteria that specifically address documentation. The ANA has specifically stated that nursing documentation is an important skill that every nurse is expected to develop and use. The ANA *1991 Standards of Clinical Nursing Practice* are listed in the Figure 1-1. I have added italics to emphasize documentation standards.

State Board of Nursing

Each state has a State Board of Nursing, which is empowered to ensure that nursing is practiced within the scope of the law. The State Board of Nursing is generally created

Figure 1-1 continued from previous page.

3. The plan reflects current nursing practice.
4. *The plan is documented.*
5. The plan provides for continuity of care.

Standard V. Implementation
THE NURSE IMPLEMENTS THE INTERVENTIONS IDENTIFIED IN THE PLAN OF CARE.

Measurement Criteria
1. Interventions are consistent with the established plan of care.
2. Interventions are implemented in a safe and appropriate manner.
3. *Interventions are documented.*

Standard VI. Evaluation
THE NURSE EVALUATES THE CLIENT'S PROGRESS TOWARD ATTAINMENT OF OUTCOMES.

Measurement Criteria
1. Evaluation is systematic and ongoing.
2. *The client's responses to interventions are documented.*
3. The effectiveness of interventions is evaluated in relation to outcomes.
4. Ongoing assessment data are used to revise diagnosis, outcomes, and the plan of care, as needed.
5. *Revisions in diagnoses, outcomes, and the plan of care are documented.*
6. The client, significant others, and health care providers are involved in the evaluation process, when appropriate.[5]

under state law to administer and enforce the Nurse Practice Act, which defines what constitutes the practice of nursing and explains licensure procedures. Laws differ in each state so it is important for the nurse to be familiar with your state's specific law. Also created by the state codes, the Act describes discipline for failure to comply with those regulations.

Review your Nurse Practice Act for the responsibilities of your State Board. Your State Board of Nursing may be responsible for:

- Evaluating nursing education programs and approving those that meet established standards.
- Denying or withdrawing approval of nursing programs not meeting standards.
- Issuing temporary and permanent license to practice nursing.
- Renewing licenses of qualified nurses.
- Establishing standards for competency for nursing and advance nursing practice.
- Carrying out the disciplinary process when necessary.

The Georgia Code Section 43-26-3(6) defines nursing as follows:

'Practice nursing' or 'practice of nursing' means to perform for compensation or the performance for compensation of any act in the care and counsel of the ill, injured, or infirmed, and in the promotion and maintenance of health with individuals, groups, or both throughout the life span. It requires substantial specialized knowledge of the humanities, natural sciences, social sciences, and nursing theory as a basis for assessment, nursing diagnosis, planning, intervention, and evaluation.[6]

Furthermore, section 43-26-3(8)(A) through (D) states:

'Practice nursing as a registered professional nurse' means to practice nursing by performing for compensation any of the following:

(A) Assessing the health status of individuals, groups, or both throughout the life span;
(B) Establishing a nursing diagnosis;
(C) Establishing nursing goals to meet identified health care needs;
(D) Planning, implementing, and evaluating nursing care;....[7]

Georgia's Codes regulating Licensed Practical Nurses, Code 400-2.12, states the following:

(1) Practice of Licensed Practical Nursing Defined. Practice of Licensed practical nursing means the provision of services for compensation, under the supervision of a physician practicing medicine, a dentist practicing dentistry, a podiatrist practicing podiatry, or a registered nurse practicing nursing in accordance with the applicable provisions of the law, the performance of which requires the formal education and preparation necessary to qualify for the examination for licensure as a licensed practical nurse, to include maintenance of health

and prevention of illness; *assisting in the assessment, planning, implementation, and evaluation of the delivery of health services;...*[8] [emphasis added.]

As you can see, LPNs are restricted to assisting in the assessment, planning, implementation, and evaluation of patients. Because the ultimate responsibility rests with the RN, hospitals require the RN to perform the admission assessment and establish nursing diagnosis. This practice holds true even though in many hospitals LPNs have the responsibilities of team leadership. The hospital and the nurses are constrained and guided by the Nurse Practice Act of their state.

Joint Commission on Accreditation of Healthcare Organizations

JCAHO is an independent agency that reviews the procedures by which a hospital or clinic operates and accredits those facilities that meet the established standards. The hospital or clinic must request the JCAHO survey and pays the organization to complete the survey. A facility that fails to meet established standards may be denied accreditation. Accredited facilities are automatically eligible for reimbursement from Medicaid and Medicare. Nonaccredited facilities can apply for participation in Medicaid and Medicare programs, but are not guaranteed approval. Because most of the hospital's operating money comes from insurance, Medicaid, and Medicare you can see why it is important to achieve accreditation. How can you as one individual nurse help achieve accreditation? By knowing the standards for accreditation in the field of nursing and complying with them within the policies and procedures of the facility where you work. The 1993 JCAHO standards that affect documentation are listed in Figure 1-2.

Other sections of the JCAHO Accreditation Manual has a direct effect on your documentation responsibilities. These sections require specific actions and the only way to prove that you complied is to document the information. Two such areas are Patient and the Family Education and Patient Self-Determination Act (see Chapter 4.)

State and Federal Government

State and federal governments control and regulate the requirements for documentation through laws associated with Medicaid and Medicare. They require that admissions be medically necessary and provide documented reasons for admission and proof of required nursing care.

Medicaid and Medicare requirements for documentation are an image of those required by the State Board of Nursing, JCAHO, and the ANA. Failure to meet those requirements could mean that Medicare or Medicaid may not reimburse the agency for that patient's care.

Two federal laws that affect nursing documentation are the Consolidated Omnibus Reconciliation Act of 1985 (COBRA) and the Patient Self-Determination Act of 1990. COBRA is designed to prevent hospitals from "dumping" or inappropriately transferring a patient who has no insurance or inadequate insurance. The hospital must screen the patient to determine whether there is an emergency medical condition or whether the patient is in active labor. In either case, the patient must be treated within the capabilities and resources of the staff and facility. The patient cannot be transferred unless the patient requests transfer or the physician makes written

---

Figure 1-2: JCAHO 1993 Nursing Standards

NC.1
Patients receive care based on a documented assessment of their needs.

NC.1.1 Each patient's need for nursing care related to his/her admission is assessed by a registered nurse.

NC.1.1.1 The assessment is conducted either at the time of admission or within a time frame preceding or following admission that is specified in hospital policy.

NC.1.1.2 Aspects of data collection may be delegated by the registered nurse.

NC.1.1.3 Needs are reassessed when warranted by the patient's condition.

NC.1.2 Each patient's assessment includes consideration of biophysical, psychosocial, environmental, self-care, educational, and discharge planning factors.

NC.1.2.1 When appropriate, data from the patient's significant other(s) are included in the assessment.

NC.1.3 Each patient's nursing care is based on identified nursing diagnoses and/or patient care needs and patient care standards, and is consistent with the therapies of other disciplines.

NC.1.3.1 The patient and/or significant other(s) are involved in the patient's care as appropriate.

NC.1.3.2 Nursing staff members collaborate, as appropriate, with physicians and other clinical disciplines in making decisions regarding each patient's need for nursing care.

NC.1.3.3 In preparation for discharge, continuing care needs are assessed and referrals for such care are documented in the patient's medical record.

Continues on the following page.

Figured 1-2 continued from previous page

NC.1.3.4 The patient's medical record includes documentation of
NC.1.3.4.1 the initial assessments and reassessments;
NC.1.3.4.2 the nursing diagnoses and/or patient care needs;
NC.1.3.4.3 the interventions identified to meet the patient's nursing care needs;
NC.1.3.4.4 the nursing care provided;
NC.1.3.4.5 the patient's response to, and the outcomes of, the care provided; and
NC.1.3.4.6 the abilities of the patient and/or, as appropriate, his/her significant other(s) to manage continuing care needs after discharge.
NC.1.3.5 Nursing care data related to patient assessments, the nursing diagnoses and/or patient needs, nursing interventions, and patient outcomes are permanently integrated into the clinical information system (for example, the medical record).
NC.1.3.5.1 Nursing care data can be identified and retrieved from the clinical information system.[9]

certification using available information that the medical benefits of the transfer outweighs the risks to the patient on or during transfer. The receiving facility must have available space and qualified personnel and be able to provide appropriate treatment. The transfer must then be completed using qualified personnel with appropriate transportation and life support equipment.

The Patient Self-Determination Act is designed to ensure that all patients are informed of their rights to make their own health care decisions regarding advanced directives. Advance directives include living wills and durable powers of attorney. A living will allows the competent patient to express his or her wishes concerning extraordinary treatment in a written format. A living will becomes effective when a patient is terminally ill and incompetent and has no reasonable chance of recovery. Durable power of attorney enables a competent person to designate another person to act in the patient's behalf if the patient should become incompetent. In this event, the designated person can make decisions regarding medical treatment. These advance directives, when available, originate from state laws. The federal Patient Self-Determination Act ensures that patients are informed of their rights under state laws. Because state laws vary, advance directives drawn up in one state may not be honored, in part or full, in another state.

Special Practice Groups

Special practice groups, such as nurses working in special care areas, nurse anesthetists, nurse midwives, and other specialists, must address other documentation standards.

These standards, not addressed here, are set by the professional organizations of those groups.

Agency Policies and Procedures

Each agency has its own policies and procedures under which you are expected to operate. The agency's standards can be stricter but not more lenient than those set up by agencies regulating the practice of nursing, accreditation, or reimbursement.

Rules regulating practices such as completion of an admission assessment are made based on area of admission. An assessment on a general medical-surgical ward may need to be completed within eight hours, whereas assessment on admission to the coronary care unit may need to be completed within one hour. Your agency will designate the form of documentation you will use, the approved abbreviation list, frequency of documentation entries, and types of forms used, among other things. You will be expected to know your agency's policies and procedures.

Most facilities have an approved list of abbreviations. The abbreviations you learn in school are used <u>almost</u> universally, but they may not be approved at all facilities. As you start to document, be sure that the abbreviations you use are on the facility-approved list, if one is established. In the past, JCAHO require a facility-approved abbreviation list, but it has removed that requirement. If your facility does not have an approved list, be very careful when using abbreviations. What can seem logical when first written may be confusing to others and lead to errors or inability to decipher now or in the future.

Summary

This chapter has emphasized the following key points:

1. Documentation is required to meet patient needs, your needs, and the needs of the institution.
2. The first reason to document is to provide high-quality patient care by communicating

important patient information to the rest of the health care team.

3. Documentation also describes the following: communication between health care team members, care provided, outcomes of care provided, and patient teaching. Documentation meets other needs, such as legal, coordination of care, DRG assignment, reimbursement, continuing education, research, and continuous quality improvement.

4. It is important to document nursing tasks such as giving medications, performing treatments, teaching patients, and obtaining expected outcomes.

5. The ANA sets standards for registered nurses that govern how nurses should practice.

6. State legislatures create the State Boards of Nurses and the Nurse Practice Acts. The Nurse Practice Act defines what constitutes the practice of nursing.

7. The JCAHO accredits those agencies that meet the established standards.

8. Agencies' policies and procedures are the local standards that you must meet when you document.

References

1. American Nurses' Association. (1980). *Nursing: A Social Policy Statement.* © Washington: Author. Reprinted with permission.
2. From *Webster's Third New International Dictionary.* © 1986 by Merriam-Webster Inc., publisher of the Merriam-Webster ® dictionaries. Reprinted with permission.
3. Feutz-Harter, S. (1989). Documentation Principles and Pitfalls. *Journal of Nursing Administration, 19* (12), 7–9.
4. Butler, P. (1991). The Nursing Shortage: The Legal Impact on Documentation. *The Journal Of Continuing Education in Nursing, 22*(5), 189–191.
5. American Nurses' Association. (1991). *Standards of Clinical Nursing Practice,* © Washington: Author. Reprinted with permission.
6. Georgia Board of Nursing. (1990). *Georgia Board of Nursing: Georgia Registered Professional Nurse Practice Act.* ©, The Michie Company, Charlottesville, VA. Reprinted with permission.
7. Georgia Board of Nursing. (1990). *Georgia Board of Nursing Georgia Registered Professional Nurse Practice Act.* ©, The Michie Company, Charlottesville, VA. Reprinted with permission.

8. Georgia Board of Practical Nursing. *(1989).Georgia Board of Practical Nursing: Georgia Practical Nurse Practice Act.* ©, The Michie Company, Charlottesville, VA. Reprinted with permission.
9. Joint Commission on Accreditation of Healthcare Organizations. (1993). *Accreditation Manual for Hospitals, Volume I Standards.* © , Oakbrook Terrance, IL: Author. Reprinted with permission.

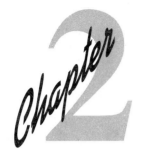

Nursing Process and Nursing Diagnosis

Chapter 2

Objectives

The learner will be able to:
1. List the components of the nursing process.
2. Explain how the nursing process is used in documentation.
3. Define nursing diagnosis.
4. Identify a correctly written NANDA diagnosis.

The nursing process is a responsibility of each nurse practicing professional nursing. The ANA's 1991 *Standards of Clinical Nursing Practice* clearly defines your responsibilities for documentation in relationship to the nursing process and patient care. Nurses are empowered and are expected to make nursing diagnosis(es) as they care for their patients by the 1980 ANA *Nursing: A Social Policy Statement*, Nurse Practice Act, and JCAHO standards.

This chapter reviews both the nursing process and the North American Nursing Diagnosis Association's (NANDA) Nursing Diagnoses. We will explore the components of the nursing process and their relationship to documentation. You were probably introduced to the nursing process in one of your very first nursing classes. If not, please refer to your nursing fundamental or medical-surgical textbooks for a more in-depth discussion of the nursing process history and its components. If you have not reviewed the NANDA Nursing Diagnoses and the use of them, please refer to these books as well.

Nursing Process

Name the five components of the nursing process. Did you say assessment, analysis (nursing diagnosis), planning, intervention (implementation), and evaluation? Did you use expected outcomes as one of your components? An expected outcome is listed as a separate standard in the ANA's *1991 Standard of Clinical Nursing Practice*,[1] but is not usually listed as a separate component in most literature about nursing process. Most have addressed expected outcomes as part of the planning phase of the process. In the future, you may see expected outcomes listed as a separate component in the nursing process.

This chapter presents the components of the nursing process as separate units. In reality, of course, the whole process is intertwined and cannot always be separated so cleanly.

The nursing process is a method to organize the nurse's thought processes to ensure that the patient's needs are addressed properly. The patient can be identified as an individual, family, group, or society. Think about organizing yourself for a day of classes. When you are able to maintain your "normal" routine, things run more smoothly and it is easier to address problems. On the days you get "off on the wrong foot," everything seems to fall apart. The nursing process is the framework for getting "off on the right foot" with your patient. By systematically approaching the patient and his/her problems you quickly establish a clinical relationship, save time, decrease hospitalization time, decrease patient discomfort, enhance time management, and improve productivity.

Nursing process includes the organized assessment of the patient, anaylsis and diagnosis of the problem(s), determination of expected outcomes, a plan to achieve the expected outcomes, implementation of the plan, and evaluation of the effectiveness of your actions and the patient's actions. This process cannot be performed in a vacuum by the nurse alone. You may obtain information and responses from the patient, significant others, acquaintances, law enforcement agencies, emergency medical personnel, other staff members, doctors, roommates, old medical records, laboratory data, and medical alert tags. As your career develops, you will learn that everyone on the hospital staff can provide important information about a patient. I have gained valuable information from the cleaning staff who have learned useful tidbits from patients as they clean the room. Listen to everyone as you do your job.

Assessment

The first step of the nursing process is assessment, the systematic approach to data collection. Each patient care area, such as a hospital unit or home care agency, has some type of organized data collection form to assess the patient's current problems and his/her ability to address those problems. In the hospital, this form is usually referred to as the nursing admission assessment. The form varies in length, but should address biophysical, psychosocial, environmental, self-care, educational, and discharge planning factors.[2] Your initial assessment of the patient will never really be complete. The process of assessment will be ongoing as further data becomes available as you develop a relationship with the patient. Your assessment will incorporate data collected through interviewing, physical assessment, clinical testing, and medical history (chart). You will collect more information about a patient and his/her life as the clinical relationship expands. You will continuously ask or look for additional data as diagnoses are defined. It is not that you have been incomplete in your initial assessment; rather, new information leads to new questions.

Analysis (Nursing Diagnosis)

Once you have collected the data, you must organize that information and define the patient's problems. This definition is your nursing diagnosis. Nursing diagnoses are those problems that a nurse can treat. A nursing diagnosis can address either a high-risk for or actual problem. Unlike the medical diagnosis, the nursing diagnosis will usually change during the patient's hospitalization, as the patient progresses or regresses on the health continuum.

A diagnosis can be made in several ways. Some hospitals use the formalized NANDA nursing diagnoses; others use an informal statement of the problem or nursing concern. Whatever format you work with, the diagnosis should be written as a clear concise statement identifying needs for nursing care. Your diagnosis must indicate a need for nursing care (patient response or patient problem), *not* a nursing task. Which of the following are *needs* for nursing care and which are nursing *tasks*?

- Skin care
- High-risk for infection
- Ambulation
- Never had surgery before
- Vital signs

If you identified skin care, ambulation, and vital signs as nursing tasks, you were correct. Nursing tasks are those interventions you do for a patient. High-risk for infection and the fact that a patient has never before had surgery are situations that require nursing skills to manage. The needs for nursing care, arising from the patient's response or problem, are your nursing diagnoses. After the diagnosis is made, the nurse must validate it, by talking with the patient and/or his family.

Expected Outcomes

Once the diagnosis has been validated, the goal(s) or expected outcomes of this hospitalization are set by the health care team and the patient. It is very important that you and the patient agree about the expected outcome. If you do not, the patient will probably be "noncompliant" or act in a way that may cause harm or prolong recovery. If a patient expects to go on a hiking trip to the mountains two weeks after a hysterectomy, the expected outcome may be jeopardized. The patient needs to be instructed on her level of activity after the surgery to prevent later complications. She will then need to establish priorities and either postpone the hiking trip or the surgery. You need to provide the information, but she needs to make the decision.

Expected outcomes must be measurable, realistic, and attainable. There must be a time set to reach the goal(s) so that you can evaluate the effectiveness of your plan and revise the plan if necessary. A realistic expected outcome considers the patient's prior capabilities and current situation. For example, a patient should not be told that he or she will be able to hike after hospitalization if before surgery he or she could only get to the mailbox because of emphysema. Finally, closely related to a realistic goal is the attainment of the goal. The goal must be attainable when available resources are considered. Expecting a homeless person to maintain a low-salt diet is unrealistic. This person is more concerned with getting any food, let alone low-salt food.

Plan of Care

After you and the patient have set the expected outcomes (goals), you must decide how to reach those expectations. This is called your plan of care or care plan. An individualized documented plan of care is necessary for each patient.[3]

The nursing profession is currently in a period of change regarding how to develop a patient plan of care. In the past, JCAHO required a care plan based on the educational care plan model. This approach always posed a problem because a formally written care plan was usually the last thing a busy nurse addressed. The care plans used in the hospital were first used in nursing education to teach students how to care for specific problems. Nurses thought that writing the plan in detail used valuable time better spent at the bedside. After many years of experience and discussion of the issue, *JCAHO has dropped the requirement for a separate nursing care plan. They still require the use of the nursing process and, therefore, a plan of care. Individual facilities are just now deciding how to address the documentation of care plans within requirements set by laws, professional organizations, and other regulatory agencies. Today a variety of formats are used.*

Regardless of this controversy, you still must develop some plan of care that is individualized for each patient and documented within the guidelines established by your institution. Just as you make a Christmas list to plan your shopping day, finances, and return time, you must plan to meet the patient's needs during the hospitalization. You must decide what interventions are necessary to move the patient from admission to discharge in the best possible condition, in the shortest time, and at the least expense.

Implementation

Once the plan has been established, it must be implemented. This is the step in the nursing process in which you provide hands-on care and teaching. Implementation helps you and the patient reach the expected outcomes established earlier.

Evaluation

During evaluation, the next phase, you decide whether the patient did or will not reach the expected outcomes. Evaluation is an interactive process in which you and the patient decide whether:

- The plan is appropriate.
- Changes need to be made.
- New information is necessary.
- The diagnosis is correct.

The evaluation is made by comparing the patient's current condition with the condition at admission or whenever the problem developed. You also need to compare the patient's status with the established expected outcomes to decide whether the patient is making progress towards the established goals. You may also uncover a new diagnosis that must be resolved before addressing the original diagnosis. During the evaluation phase, it is determined whether the problem has been resolved and whether the patient is no longer at risk. Once the evaluation has been made, you may reenter the nursing process at any of the preceding phases.

Nursing Process in Practice

The components of the nursing process are intertwined throughout the patient's hospital stay. Every time you do an intervention you are looking at the patient and evaluating the response(s). You add or delete interventions to the plan based on that evaluation. You gather and validate additional information about the patient's abilities, environment, and health with each interaction.

As a nurse you use the nursing process to provide organized high-quality patient care and meet your professional responsibilities. The nursing process is the framework of the professional nurse's practice. You use the nursing process to your patient's benefit.

Exercise 2-1

Indicate which component of the nursing process is addressed by the following forms.

FORMS	NURSING PROCESS COMPONENT
1. Nursing Admission Assessment (Initial data collection regarding the patient's biophysical, psychosocial, environmental, self-care, educational, and discharge planning factors.)	1._____
2. Medication Administration Record (Form to record medicines the patient is given, times administered, and who gave them.)	2._____
3. Intake and Output (Form to record all fluids a patient has ingested and all liquid output or drainage.)	3._____
4. Activity of Daily Living Flow Sheet (Form designed to document routine care given to patients.)	4._____
5. Progress notes (Nursing notes about the patient's day-to-day condition.)	5._____

Exercise 2-1 Answers

1. Nursing Admission Assessment is the <u>assessment</u> part of the nursing process. During the admission assessment you may also evaluate care that was provided before hospitalization.
2. Medication Administration Record is part of the <u>implementation</u> component of the nursing process. You are providing nursing care, medication administration, and documentation of the same.
3. I & O is from the <u>implementation</u> and <u>evaluative</u> components. You document fluids given to and the amount of drainage from the patient and assess the patient's fluid balance, making sure that the patient is not dehydrated, overloaded, or developing kidney failure.
4. Activity of Daily Living Flow Sheet is used to document the <u>implementation</u> component of the nursing process.
5. Progress notes are used in <u>all components</u> of the nursing process.

Exercise 2-2

To help you understand how progress notes are used for all nursing process components review the following notes. Indicate what component of the nursing process you are reviewing.

1. 29-year-old Caucasian male admitted to room 2B via stretcher from ED. Admitted to Orthopedic Service under Dr. Riley's care with diagnosis of fractured right ankle. _____
2. No known drug allergies (NKDA) _____
3. HOB elevated 90 degrees, O_2 per nasal cannula at 2 L/min, BP 180/100 P 108 R 24. _____
4. Demerol 100 mg IM given in left ventrogluteal region.... _____
5. Fluid volume deficit related to decreased oral intake _____
6. Active bowel sounds in all quadrants, abdomen soft and nontender, passing flatus, denies gas pains. _____
7. Started patient instruction on insulin injection technique, shown video "Giving Yourself Insulin Injection," demonstrated techniques of 1) handling needle and syringe, 2) preparing insulin bottle, 3) extracting insulin, 4) skin prep, and 5) injection of medication. Patient did well with steps 1, 2, and 4, maintained good technique without difficulty. _____

8. Pain will be controlled on oral medications by 3rd day post-op. _____
9. Assess breathe sounds and breathing patterns q4h and monitor ABGs as ordered.
_____

Are you comfortable with you choices? Let's see if we agree.

Exercise 2-2 Answers

1. <u>Assessment</u>: The typical opening line of an admission summary written after the Nursing Admission Assessment is completed.
2. <u>Assessment</u>: Part of the information documented in the admission summary. It is extremely important to ensure that allergy information is documented adequately. Allergy histories need to be documented in the following places: admission assessment, admission summary, Kardex, medication administration record, front of chart. Allergy histories are also found on colored arm bands, pre-op check lists, and transfer summaries. Be sure to follow protocols for notification of pharmacy of any allergies.
3. <u>Implementation</u>: The documentation of nursing care that you have completed. <u>Assessment or evaluation</u>: Vital signs are monitored to assess the effects of treatment to or physiologic conditions on the patient.
4. <u>Implementation</u>: Care provided to the patient.
5. <u>Nursing Diagnosis</u>: A formal NANDA nursing diagnosis. "Fluid volume deficit" is a statement of the problem. "Related to decreased oral intake" is a statement that declares where the problem comes from.
6. <u>Assessment or Evaluation</u>: If this statement is part of an admission summary it would be an assessment. If the same note is seen on a postoperative chart of a patient who had abdominal surgery, it would be an evaluative statement.
7. <u>Implementation</u>: Statement about patient education or implementation of a care plan to teach self-care to a patient diagnosed as "insulin dependent diabetic." <u>Evaluation</u>: The note is also evaluative because it discusses how the patient did when he tried to administer insulin. To be complete, the note should state the patient's attempt to give an injection to an orange or himself and requirements for further teaching.

8. <u>Expected Outcomes</u>: "Pain will be controlled" is a specific statement about outcome. Stating that the patient will have pain controlled with oral medications by 3rd day post-op provides a marker to evaluate your patient's condition.

9. <u>Planning</u>: All three items are nursing care to be done for a patient. If the tasks were completed, this list would be implementation.

Progress notes are the one form of nursing documentation that documents all phases of the nursing process. Other forms were developed to improve and streamline the documentation process. These supportive forms usually address one or two components of the nursing process. The major exception to this general guideline is that ICU and Newborn Nurseries often use complex flow sheets to meet most of their documentation needs.

The nursing process is a very integral component of your nursing practice. You need to understand how to use the nursing process to help you provide high-quality patient care. Documentation is one method to evaluate your use of the nursing process.

NANDA Nursing Diagnoses

The second component of the nursing process is analysis where nursing diagnoses are defined. The ANA has officially adopted the NANDA diagnoses as the official system of nursing diagnosis.[4] We will briefly review the NANDA's system.

NANDA's definition of nursing diagnosis is as follows:

> A nursing diagnosis is a clinical judgment about an individual, family, or community response to actual or potential health problems/life processes which provides the basis for definitive therapy toward achievement of outcomes for which the nurse is accountable.[5]

A nursing diagnosis can identify an actual or high-risk for problem related to one of nine different patterns of human response. Actual problems identify currently existing health problem(s). High-risk for problems are those in which a potential problem is identified but has not yet developed. The nine human response patterns used for the nursing diagnosis taxonomy are the following:

- Exchange
- Communicating
- Relating
- Valuing
- Choosing
- Moving
- Perceiving
- Knowing
- Feeling

Under each of the human response patterns are many nursing diagnoses that could potentially be used with patients with a wide range of medical diagnoses.

Writing a nursing diagnosis starts with the identification of the patient's response to the current health problem. You then need to identify what that response is related to. For example, your patient is admitted with the medical diagnosis of asthma. After completing the assessment, you find one of the patient's responses to the asthma is activity intolerance. The activity intolerance is caused by dyspnea and fatigue. To generate a nursing diagnosis, combine the human response with the cause using the phrase *related to*. Your final diagnosis reads *activity intolerance related to dyspnea and fatigue*.

The following guidelines should be used when writing nursing diagnosis:

1. Focus on the patient's response.
2. The first part of the diagnosis identifies the human response.
3. *Related to* is always the connecting phase between the two parts of the nursing diagnosis.

4. The second part of the diagnosis identifies the factors that are causing or contributing to the problem.
5. The related factor must be expressed in a format that can be changed by nursing care.
6. Defining characteristics may be added to the first two components of the statement using the phrase *characterized by* or *evident by* as connectors.
7. Make the diagnostic statement as clear as possible by using concise statements.

When writing nursing diagnosis:

8. Do not identify a nurse's problem, needs, or task.
9. Do not assign blame.
10. Do not make value judgments.
11. Do not use a single symptom or clue as the human response part of the diagnosis.
12. Do not say the same thing with both parts of the diagnosis.
13. Do not use a medical diagnosis as a component of the nursing diagnosis.

Exercise 2-3:

Review the following nursing diagnostic statements and decide whether they are correct. If they are improperly written, decide which of the guidelines needs to be followed and rewrite the statement correctly.

1. Gas exchange, impaired due to altered blood flow.
   Correct/Incorrect_____

   _____

2. Communication, impaired: verbal related to refusal to learn English.
   Correct/Incorrect_____

   _____

3. Pneumonia related to trauma.
   Correct/Incorrect _____

   _____

4. Parenting, altered related to lack of available role model.
   Correct/Incorrect _____

   _____

5. Tissue integrity, impaired related to poor nursing care.
   Correct/Incorrect _____

   _____

6. High-risk for infection related to invasive procedures.
   Correct/Incorrect _____

   _____

Let's see if we agree on the answers.

Exercise 2-3 Answers

1. Incorrect. Gas exchange, impaired <u>due to</u> altered blood flow. Guideline #3 Correction: Gas exchange, impaired <u>related to</u> altered blood flow.
2. Incorrect. Communication, impaired: verbal related to <u>refusal to learn English</u>. Guideline #10 Correction: Communication, impaired: verbal related to <u>inability to speak English</u>.
3. Incorrect. <u>Pneumonia</u> related to trauma. Guideline #13 Correction: <u>Airway clearance, ineffective</u> related to trauma.
4. Correct.
5. Incorrect. Tissue integrity, impaired related to <u>poor nursing care</u>. Guideline #9 Correction: Tissue integrity, impaired related to <u>impaired physical mobility</u>.
6. Correct.

How can you use a NANDA Nursing Diagnosis to guide the documentation of patient care? The Nursing Diagnosis identifies a specific problem that is explicitly described. The human response, or first part of the diagnosis, identifies the concern. The second part identifies the expected cause. Both parts of the diagnosis must be addressed in documentation.

For example, let's look at diagnosis #5, tissue integrity, impaired related to impaired physical mobility. You will need to address the wound or area of skin breakdown including the appearance, how well it is healing, and the treatments to improve healing. You must also discuss the impaired physical mobility. What is being done to prevent further problems and improve mobility? Changes in ability to move without help should also be noted.

Summary

This chapter has emphasized the following key points:

1. The nursing process is the official framework of professional nursing.
2. The five components of the nursing process are assessment, analysis (nursing diagnosis), planning, intervention, and evaluation. Expected outcomes are part of planning.
3. Assessment is the collection of the patient database.
4. Nursing diagnosis is the definition of the patient's problems that require nursing care. Nursing diagnosis must be validated with the patient to prevent wasted time or effort.
5. Expected outcomes are the goals for nursing care.
6. Planning involves decision making about what must be done to reverse the identified problem.
7. Intervention is the hands-on nursing care.
8. Evaluation is the process of deciding whether the nursing care is effective and whether the problem is resolved or the patient is still at risk.
9. Use of the nursing process must be documented on several different forms including

the following: Nursing Admission Assessment, Medication Administration Records, Activity of Daily Living Flow Sheets, I & O, and Progress Notes.

10. A NANDA Nursing Diagnosis is written in two parts. Part one identifies the human response to the problem. The part two identifies the factor that the problem is related to.

11. Both parts are connected by the phase *related to*.

References

1. American Nurses Association. (1991). *Standards of Clinical Nursing Practice*. Washington: Author.

2. Joint Commission on Accreditation of Healthcare Organizations. (1993). *Accreditation Manual for Hospitals, Volume 1 Standards*. Oakbrook Terrance, Ill.: Author, 79–80.

3. American Nurses Association. (1991). *Standards of Clinical Nursing Practice*. Washington: Author.

4. Lang, N.M., & Gibbie, K. (1988). Nursing Taxonomy: NANDA and ANA Joint Venture toward ICD-10CM. In R. Carroll-Johnson (Ed.). *Classification of Nursing Diagnosis, Proceeding of the Eighth Conference*. (pp. 11–17). Philadelphia: J. B. Lippincott Company.

5. Reprinted with permission from North American Nursing Diagnosis Association. (1992). *NANDA Nursing Diagnosis: Definitions and Classification 1992–1993*, © Philadelphia: NANDA.

Notes:

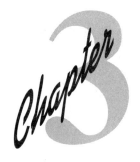

Documentation Formats

The learner will be able to:
1. Identify the different formats of nursing documentation.

Several documentation systems are currently used in nursing. Each has its own advantages and disadvantages for helping the nurse document patient care. The Nursing Department of each hospital or agency has to decide which system best meets professional responsibilities and patient needs. As a student, you need to know that there is more than one way to document patient care. You may even find different documentation systems within the facility in which you complete your clinical experiences. Because documentation plays such a vital role in nursing and is so time-consuming, nursing departments are constantly reviewing their systems and making changes. This chapter introduces you to four of the most common systems of documentation: source-oriented, problem-oriented, process-oriented, and a combination of the three. These systems differ in their organization. Source-oriented systems rely on the practitioner as the source of the data. Problem-oriented systems revolve around the nursing problems. The newest system the process-oriented system, revolves around the nursing process. This system allows for broader identification of problems that concern the nurse.

Nursing documentation systems consist of a combination of flow sheets, graphic records, and narrative notes. These forms are designed in many ways and are used differently. No matter how the system operates, it must meet the requirements as identified in Chapter 1.

Source-Oriented: Narrative

Narrative documentation, a source-oriented system, is the oldest system of documentation used by the medical/nursing profession. Still widely used today by many professions in the health care system, narrative documentation is structured so that the content of each progress note is totally determined by its author.

The nurse is given no guidance as to what each note should contain. (S)he must learn through experience and decide what is important to document and to develop his/her own system to decide organization to complete a note. Notes are written in chronological order. The free form of narrative notes makes this format usable in any type of clinical situation.

The free form can produce notes that are fragmented and noninformative. For example consider the following note that an evening nurse routinely wrote about each patient:

> PM care done.
> Regular diet, ate 3/4.
> Up in chair.
> Visitors in
> HS care done
> Quiet evening

This basic note would sometimes be supplemented with an occasional note about a patient problem. Even though this note met the documentation requirements when it was written 20 years ago, it did not say anything; it only met the institution's requirement to document on each patient's record on every shift. The note demonstrates an inherent problem with the narrative form of documentation: No information was given because nurses did not receive any direction about what should be documented. On the other hand, a narrative note can be too wordy, making it difficult to pick out patient trends and problems. In addition, this form of charting often takes longer to complete because the lack of structure and guidelines encourages rambling, nonspecific narrative entries.

Some facilities separate each group of professional notes from each other. Nurses document on nursing notes, doctors document on doctors progress notes, and so on. This organization of notes requires the reader to look through the chart to obtain all the required information. In other facilities, all professionals document on the same sheets of paper, but indicate their profession.

Example 3-1: Narrative Format

The Example 3-1 is a narrative format nursing note.

11/19/92 0328	Patient complaining of substernal, nonradiating chest pain that started 20 minutes ago. Denies dyspnea or nausea. Skin cool and damp, color dusky. BP 90/56 P 112 R 24. HOB placed in high Fowler's position, O_2 put on at 2 L/min/nasal cannula. ————
0332	Called Dr. Smith and advised of all information in 0328 note, see doctors orders. ————
0345	Given SL nitroglycerine 1/150 gr at 0333 repeated at 0338 and 0343 without relief. Vitals were 0333 BP 90/48 P 114 R 25, 0338 88/46 P 117 R 25. 0343 BP 88/46 P 118 R 25. Restless and rubbing chest saying "Feels like an elephant is sitting on my chest." ————
0346	Recalled Dr. Smith and advised of changes and actions noted in 0345 note, see doctors orders. ———— *S. Esteves RN*

Obviously, this particular story continues, but we will stop here.

Problem-Oriented: SOAP(IE)(IER)

SOAP noting was developed in the 1960s by Dr. Lawrence Weed for use by doctors. In this problem-oriented system of documentation, each identified problem is charted as a separate note. Nurses have adopted the SOAP format of documentation in many clinical areas of nursing. SOAP has four parts: 1) database, 2) problem list, 3) care plan, and 4) progress notes. The database (assessment) was once a feature only of the SOAP format of documentation, but today assessments are an essential component of all systems of documentation.

The database is all of the information collected about the patient during the nursing admission assessment. Based on the assessment, the problem list is developed, which includes all actual and high-risk problems for nursing diagnoses. These problems must be numbered and priorities established. The care plan is a record of your plan to treat or help the patient adapt to the identified problems. Progress notes are written to document explicit information about the patient, care rendered, problems developed, and other important data.

The term SOAP(IE)(IER) is an acronym that stands for the following:

S: Subjective information that the patient provides. Example: "I have been having chest pains for the last 20 minutes." Or, has had green drainage from leg abrasion for the last three days before admission. Denies fever, foul odor, or pain.

O: Objective information is information collected by the nurse through physical assessment, observation, monitoring, or laboratory data or information obtained from anyone other than the patient.

A: Assessment is the (re)statement of the nursing diagnosis and identification of progress toward resolving the problem. Evaluative statements can be made here, but data must be included in either the S or O to support that statement.

P: Plans are what you plan to do now or in the future for this patient and this particular problem. These plans must not counteract orders or plans made by the doctor or other health care professionals.

The original SOAP notes stopped here, but as SOAP notes were used more and more, the following areas were added.

I: Interventions are those actions that you as a nurse will do or direct others to do to help the patient attain an optimum level of health.

E: Evaluation is an assessment of whether the above interventions are having the desired effect or if the plan of care must be revised.

R: Revisions are the changes you make to the care plan based on the above evaluation.

SOAP noting allows the nurse to address specific problems in an organized manner. The structure of these notes guide the nurse's thoughts to include the patient's thoughts or concerns, data the nurse has about that problem, assessment, planning of care, evaluation, and revision. (Can you see the steps of the nursing process in the SOAP note form?)

This format is difficult to use when there is a fast-paced change in the patient's condition, or when the problem list is not used or kept current. Routine care is difficult to document if flow sheets are not used.

SOAP notes are extremely difficult to work with for nurses who have 8 to 12 hours of constant contact with a patient. They are best used in clinical situations where nurses make summary notes for a day, week, or month at a time.

A SOAP note would look like the one in Example 3-2.

Example 3-2: SOAP Format

11/19/92 S: "I'm having pain in my chest." Pain is substernal nonradiating.
0350   20 Minutes in duration, denies dyspnea or nausea.————————
          O: Skin cool and damp, color dusky. VS at 0333 BP 90/56
          P 112 R 24. Respirations nonlabored and regular. Placed in
          high Fowler's position, O_2 on 2 L/min/nasal cannula, called and
          advised Dr. Smith of above. See orders. SL nitroglycerine
          given at 0333, 0338, and 0343 with no relief of pain. VS at
          0338 BP 88/46 P 117 R 25 and 0343 BP 88/46 P 118
          R 25. After nitroglycerine restless and rubbing chest with a
          clenched fist stating "Feels like an elephant is sitting on my
          chest." Recalled Dr. Smith at 0345 and advised of changes noted
          above, orders received. ————————————————————
          A: Pain related to chest pain unrelieved by nitroglycerine and O_2.
          P: Transfer to ICU, give report to ICU staff, call family and
          advise of change of condition.———————— *F. Honn RN*

SOAPIER notes would read like Example 3-3.

Example 3-3: SOAPIER Format

11/19/92 S: "I'm having pain in my chest." Pain is substernal nonradiating.
0350   20 minutes in duration, denies dyspnea or nausea.
          O: Skin cool and damp, color dusky. BP 90/56 P 112 R 24.
          Respirations nonlabored and regular. ————————————
          A: Pain related to chest pain.————————————————
          P: Place in high Fowler's position, O_2 at 2 L/min/nasal cannula.
          Keep staff member with patient, continue monitoring vital signs,
          and call Dr. Smith. ————————————————————
          I: Called and advised Dr. Smith of above information, orders
          received. O_2 in place, in high Fowler's, SL nitroglycerine given
          at 0333, 0338, and 0343.————————————————————
          E: VS were at 0338 BP 88/46 P 117 R 25 and at 0343 BP 88/46
          P 118 R 25. Restless and rubbing chest with a clenched fist
          stating "Feels like an elephant is sitting on my chest."————
          R: Recall Dr. Smith and advise of above changes and actions.
          ——————————————————————— *F. Honn RN*

Process-Oriented: Charting by Exception

Charting by Exception (CBE)[1] is a form of process-oriented nursing documentation developed by nurses specifically to meet their needs regarding documentation and time usage. The main thrust is to document only those conditions that deviate from the patient's normal status.

The three key components of the CBE system are:

1. Flow sheets that set assessment parameters and highlight significant findings.
2. The use of Standards of Nursing Practice as a guide for documentation.
3. Documentation forms placed at the bedside.

Standards of Nursing Practice, which describe what is considered normal, are developed and used to guide nurses in assessing the patient. If the patient meets that established norm, then documentation is completed with a check mark and the nurse's initials or signature. If the patient falls outside the norm, then further documentation is required, beginning with marking the flow sheet with an asterisk. The asterisk refers the reader to a nurse's progress notes where further elaboration is made.

A typical standard could read like the following taken from an obstetrical/gynecological assessment flow sheet:

Neuro: Alert, oriented to ppt, sensation intact, no visual disturbances, no h/a, DTRs 1-2+ bilat., no clonus.[2]

A finding of a patient who is confused, after being alert and oriented, would be a deviation that would require a progress note made in the SOAP(IER) format.

The CBE format of documentation uses flow sheets to streamline and expedite nursing documentation. The flow sheets are the focus of this charting system and include nursing/physician order flow sheets, graphic record, nurses notes, patient teaching record, and patient discharge note.

Process-Oriented: Focus Charting™

Focus Charting is another process-oriented nursing documentation system developed by nurses to meet their specific needs. Focus Charting is a patient-centered approach to documentation that directs the organization of progress notes. Because it is user friendly, Focus Charting is being used by more and more nursing departments as the preferred system of documentation. The notes are organized to develop, support, and direct a new nurse's thinking pattern. (The focus format will be used throughout the rest of this manual to illustrate examples of progress notes.)

The focus of a narrative note can be one of many different topics that the nurse must address to ensure quality care via comprehensive documentation. A focus can be any of the following topics: key phase of nursing diagnosis, patient's concern, patient's behavior, sign or symptom, acute change in patient's condition, significant event in patient care, elaboration of documentation on flow sheet, phrase indicating compliance with standards of care/hospital policy, and occasionally, a medical diagnosis.[3] Examples of a focus could include respiratory function, reflex incontinence, left leg pain, dyspnea, headache, fever, vomiting, CPR, post liver biopsy, decreased intake, change in Foley drainage, fear, self-concept disturbance, and postoperative assessment.

Points to remember about identifying a focus:

1. A focus is identified and documented in a separate column to the left of the narrative portion of the note.
2. The focus must be patient centered, not a nursing procedure. The focus should be the wound, not wound care.
3. The nursing diagnosis or focus must be identified the same way throughout the hospital stay to allow the reader to track the problem. It should be identified the same way in the focus column and the care plan.
4. The focus is a sign or symptom that you are monitoring before finalizing a nursing or

medical diagnosis. This focus changes during the hospital stay if you formalize a nursing diagnosis.

5. A focus should indicate a nursing diagnosis or problem that nurses can treat. Recall the ANA's definition of nursing from Chapter 1: The doctor treats the fractured leg, and you treat the patient's pain and teach cast care.

6. A medical diagnosis is rarely used, but occasionally, it is used in the critical care area that has protocols for treating medical problems. Hospital policy should state which medical diagnoses are permissible.

Focus Charting uses flow sheets and narrative notes to document patient care. Flow sheets are used to document routine care. Narrative notes are separated into three columns: a column each for the date/time, focus, and narrative note, which allows the reader to quickly identify the patient's problems or nursing diagnosis.

DATE/TIME	FOCUS	PATIENT CARE NOTES
		Data
		Action
		Response

The patient care notes are broken down further into three separate areas: **D**ata, **A**ction, and **R**esponses.[4]

Data: Any information, subjective or objective, about the patient, including blood pressures, patient statements, observations of a wound, details of admission assessment, or information as reported by parents.

Action: Anything past, present, or future that you have done or will do for the patient. Actions could include elevated head of bed, call doctor, O_2 at 2 L/min, or patient teaching.

Response: How the patient responded to the medical or nursing care. Responses include lack of relief from pain or constipation, decreased dyspnea, or able to self-administer insulin.

Example 3-4 is an example of a Focus Charting nursing progress note.

Example 3-4: Focus Format

11/19/92 0328	Chest pain	D: Complaining of substernal, nonradiating chest pain that started 20 minutes ago. Denies dyspnea or nausea. Skin cool and damp, color dusky. BP 90/56 P 112 R 24.———————— A: HOB in high Fowler's. O_2 put back on at 2 L/minute/nasal cannula. Call Dr. Smith and advise of above. *G. Bass RN*
11/19/92 0346	Chest pain	D: Orders received from 0329 call to Dr. Smith. 0338 BP 88/46 P 117 R 25 and at 0343 BP 88/46 P 118 R 25.———— A: Nitroglycerine given X 3, see MAR, Recalled Dr. Smith and advised in further change in condition, orders received. R: No relief obtained from nitroglycerine. Restless and rubbing chest saying "Feels like an elephant is sitting on my chest."———————— *G. Bass RN*

If no note was written until all of these events had occurred, only one note would be necessary rather than the two shown here.

Note: In any of the examples used in this chapter, the vital signs could have been noted on flow sheets used for recording frequent vital signs. The nurse may use personal judgment for the location of documentation for a limited number of vital signs that do not fit on the graphic. You can either include them in you narrative note or use a flow sheet. This holds true only for very few sets of vital signs. If there are more than two or three sets of vital signs, they should be documented on flow sheets.

Any particular focus narrative note may include a DAR, DA, D, or R segment or any other combination. You can structure the note to meet your documentation needs. Review the following note:

Example 3-5: Focus Format (one and two segment notes)

| 12/6/92 1015 | Constipation | D: No BM, since 12/2, experiencing slight nausea and abdominal fullness. Active bowel sounds in all quadrants.——————— A: Called and advised Dr. Jones of above. MOM given at 1010. Instructed to drink 8 glasses water a day, ambulate 3-4 times a day with rest periods so as not to tire self, increase fiber in diet.——— *R. Wright LPN* |
| 12/6/92 2230 | Constipation | R: Had large BM and reports feeling much better, denies nausea.——— *D. Wilson RN* |

The focus system of nursing documentation is flexible and allows the nurse to address nursing concerns easily. The system is easy to use, and a quick review of the focus column shows the nursing concerns. Nurses must be careful to address the focus consistently between the care plan and narrative notes. To ensure proper follow-up, all nurses must review prior documentation.

Computers

Computers are not a system of documentation, but rather a method of documentation. Computers have been used for years in the business areas of the hospital and are now moving into the nursing areas. They are being used to document patient care, management reports, patient classifications, and staffing projections. Some hospitals are equipped with bedside terminals to input patient data: others have station terminals only. The information you are required to document is the same, whether you document with a pen and paper or a computer. Computers are in nursing's future, so you should expect to be working more and more with computers when you document.

Other Systems

Other systems of documentation include: CORE Documentation System, FACT Charting, PIE (Problem Identification, Interventions, and Evaluation), Outcome Documentation, and Narrative Construct. They also have their place in nursing documentation and are used in various facilities. They have their own strengths and weaknesses as documentation systems and are a variation of the four formats covered in this chapter.

Exercise 3-1

1. Identify which component applies to the following notations, S, O, A, P, I, E, or R for a SOAP note or D, A, or R for a FOCUS note.

                                                          SOAP   FOCUS

   A. Instruct on high-fiber diet.   ____   ____

   B. Foley drainage bright red with clots.   ____   ____

   C. I have this pain in my arm.   ____   ____

   D. Taught to administer inhaler.   ____   ____

   E. Teach to do sterile dressing changes.   ____   ____

   F. Reports pain now 2 on scale of 10.   ____   ____

   G. Capillary refill <3 seconds, toes warm,
      denies numbness or tingling.   ____   ____

   H. Turn, cough, and deep breathe q2h.   ____   ____

2. Document the following information in both the SOAP and FOCUS formats. Mrs. Jarvis has an NG tube that drained 300cc on the last shift, but in the last 6 hours it has drained only 50cc. She is complaining of nausea, which she hasn't had for 36 hours after the tube was placed. Has no bowel sounds, abdomen soft, passing no

flatus or belching. Tube placement checked and found to be out of place. NG tube repositioned with immediate drainage of 200cc of dark brown fluid, guaiac trace positive. Patient reports resolution of nausea. Tube placement checked; tube is in place.

A. SOAP format:

B. FOCUS format:

Exercise 3-1 Answers

1. Identify which component applies to the following notations, S, O, A, P, I, E, or R for a SOAP note or D, A, or R for a FOCUS note.

	SOAP	FOCUS
A. Instruct on high-fiber diet.	P/I	A
B. Foley drainage bright red with clots.	O	D
C. I have this pain in my arm.	S	D
D. Taught to administer inhaler.	I	A
E. Teach to do sterile dressing changes.	P	A
F. Reports pain now 2 on scale of 10.	E	R
G. Capillary refill <3 seconds, toes warm, denies numbness or tingling.	O	D
H. Turn, cough, and deep breathe q2h.	P/I	A

2. Document the following information in both the SOAP and FOCUS formats. Mrs. Jarvis has an NG tube that drained 300cc on the last shift, but in the last 6 hours it has drained only 50cc. She is complaining of nausea, which she hasn't had for 36 hours after the tube was placed. Has no bowel sounds, abdomen soft, passing no flatus or belching. Tube placement checked and found to be out of place. NG tube repositioned with immediate drainage of 200cc of dark brown fluid, guaiac trace positive. Patient reports resolution of nausea. Tube placement checked; tube is in place.

   A. SOAP Format:
   S: I'm nauseated. Denies passing flatus or belching. ———————
   O: NG drained only 50cc in last 6 hours compared to 300cc the previous 8 hours. No bowel sounds, abdomen soft. NG found to be out of place. NG repositioned, placement checked and verified in place with auscultation and positive drainage of 200cc of dark brown fluid. NG drainage guaiac trace positive. ———————
   A: Altered Nutrition: Less Than Body Requirements related to vomiting and fluid restriction. Nausea relieved. *B. Harve LPN*

Continued P: Monitor tube placement, assess nausea again in
1 hour, I & O in 2 hours. ———————*B. Harve LPN*

B. FOCUS format:

Nausea   D: Complaining of nausea, last nausea was 36 hours ago. No
bowel sounds, abdomen soft, denies passing flatus or belching. NG
drained 50cc in last 6 hours compared to 300cc in the previous 8
hours. NG out of place.————————————————————
A: NG tube repositioned, placement checked with auscultation,
placement verified. Will monitor tube placement, assess nausea in
1 hour, I & O in 2 hours. ——————————————————
R: 200cc of dark brown fluid, guaiac trace positive, obtained
immediately with tube repositioning. Nausea resolved. *K. Baird RN*

Summary

This chapter has emphasized the following key points:

1. There are many different systems of documentation, including Narrative, SOAP(IE) (IER), Charting by Exception, FOCUS, PIE, CORE, Outcome Documentation, and Narrative Construct.

2. The Narrative system is an unstructured, source-oriented documentation. Notes are written in chronological order.

3. SOAP(IE)(IER) is a problem-oriented system of documentation. The acronym stands for Subjective, Objective, Assessment, Plan, Interventions, Evaluation, and Revisions data. This system gives the nurse guidance when writing progress notes.

4. Charting by Exception, a process-oriented system of documentation, decreases documentation time by requiring the nurse to document only deviations from defined normals.

5. Focus Charting® is a process-oriented system of documentation that is patient centered. The focus is the problem/nursing

diagnosis that the nurse is addressing in the progress note.

6. A focus can be a key phase of nursing diagnosis, patient concern patient behavior, sign or symptoms, acute change in patient's condition, significant event in the patient's care, elaboration of documentation from flow sheet, phase indicating compliance with standards of care/hospital policy, and occasionally a medical diagnosis.

7. All systems now use flow sheets, graphics, and narrative notes to document patient care.

References

1. Burke, L. J. & Murphy, J. (1988). *Charting By Exception*. Media, PA: Harwal Publishing Company.
2. Boulder Community Hospital. (1992). *Ob/Gyn Assessment Flow Sheet*. Boulder, Co.: Unpublished form.
3. Lampe, S. S. (1988). *Focus Charting*™. Minneapolis: Creative Nursing Management, Inc., 18–21.
4. Lampe, S. S. (1988). *Focus Charting*™. Minneapolis: Creative Nursing Management, Inc., 23.

When and How To Document

The learner will be able to:
1. List conditions when documentation is necessary.
2. Use proper techniques in documentation.
3. Avoid the common pitfalls of documentation.

This chapter discusses when you must document to ensure quality patient care and outlines the proper techniques of nursing documentation. This information will help you develop clear, concise notes that can affect your patient care. Chapters 5 and 6 provide further discussion and examples of many of the situations presented in this chapter.

When to Document

There are some very specific times when you must document patient care/status to meet your professional responsibilities as outlined in Chapter 1. The goal is to provide quality care for the patient by communicating essential facts to health care team members and to meet other obligations that require documentary evidence.

Admission Assessment

Narrative documentation requirements begin after you complete the nursing admission assessment. The assessment is composed of individual pieces of information about the patient's life and health—past, present, and future. After completing the assessment, you organize the information and summarize it into an admission nursing note. The note contains information obtained from the assessment, physical examination, clinical data, and any other relevant data.

Information in the admission note includes time of admission, age, ethnic background, sex, occupation, room number, mode of travel to ward, accompanied by, diagnosis, doctor, service, and allergies. Also included are chief complaint, history of same, signs and symptoms (both presence and absence), vital signs, and attempts to treat before hospitalization. Identified problems, treatments begun, specimens obtained and time sent to lab, and any barriers to providing care or self-care (blindness or low IQ) must also be addressed. Finally, you must document information related to legal protection including valuables and their disposition, time doctor notified and information reported, consults sent, identified discharge planning needs, and any part of admission assessment not completed and why.[1]

> **The goal of documentation is to provide quality patient care by communicating essential facts to health care team members and to meet other obligations that require documentary evidence.**

You want to define the patient's condition on arrival to your unit or care by establishing physical or psychological condition, nursing needs, and goals (set with the patient) and to demonstrate that the patient needs to be in the hospital. While writing the admission summary, you may refer the reader to the actual care plan, thereby eliminating the need to write the information twice.

Patient's Condition

You document when the patient gets better or worse or makes no progress on the identified nursing diagnosis in a realistic amount of time. Documentation of the changes or lack of changes in the patient's condition helps all team members evaluate the effectiveness of the plan of care and make changes to the plan if required. This is the "routine" daily documentation that you do on each patient and problem.

You need to address each nursing diagnosis at prescribed intervals which are set by the nursing department's policies and procedures. The intervals of documentation depend on the patient's acuity, level of illness, and amount of nursing required.

When addressing each problem, you should identify the status of each diagnosis. Is the patient's condition improving, unchanged, or deteriorating? Can you demonstrate that the patient is getting better? How is the patient better? Worse? No change in a reasonable amount of time? Say so. You want to clearly define the patient's condition.

After identifying the patient's progress or lack of progress, appropriate changes need to be made to the care plan. Interventions may be deleted or added, or the plan may be completely revised. When the patient makes no progress, ask yourself whether the diagnosis is correct. If not, what is the correct diagnosis?

New Nursing Diagnosis

New diagnosis or problem(s), once identified, must be documented as quickly as possible. Initially, this may mean documenting a new symptom or change in behavior. As you start monitoring a new symptom, either other symptoms will follow or the problem will resolve and need no further follow-up. You want to document any new symptoms or problems quickly because the symptom may be the key to the situation, and noting it will allow the health care team to give definitive treatment. Be sure to show what measures you have taken to address the problem. What nursing interventions did you initiate in response to your evaluation of the problem?

Problem Resolved

You need to document when a problem is identified and treatment results in meeting the expected outcomes or the resolution of that problem. Your nursing note should identify the problem addressed. It should provide data that indicates that the problem is no longer active and a statement that the problem is resolved. You need to decide whether the problem still needs to be monitored and documented. You do not want to waste time documenting something that is no longer a problem, but neither do you want to neglect a problem.

Patient Education

Patients must be given information so that they can make informed decisions, know what to expect, and take care of themselves after discharge. This education of the patient and/or his/her significant others must be documented in the medical record. Often, the nursing staff explains things to the patient, but fails to document such teaching. You need to document what the patient has been taught so that others can continue any teaching that is necessary.

When documenting patient education, instructions, or counseling you need to indicate the ability of the patient to do the care, understand the information, and plan to follow through. You also need to communicate any further teaching or reinforcement requirements, the way in which evaluation of learning was completed, and plans to ensure the completion of the teaching or reinforcement. Include who was taught, the objective of the teaching session, the titles of handouts or educational programs used, and models used to demonstrate information. Pay close attention to discharge instructions when documenting.

Pre-procedure and Post-procedure

When performing a procedure, document what you did, supplies used, observations made, and the effects of that treatment. If the procedure is done by the doctor with your assistance, state which doctor did the procedure. The doctor is also responsible for documenting what was done.

Some facilities have flow sheets to document repetitive procedures, such as wound care. You will need to make pre-procedure notes on any patient undergoing an invasive procedure either on or off the unit. Pre-procedure notes should show completion of the ordered prep, the effects of the prep, education, consents signed, emotional status or concerns about the procedure, and the patient's condition at start or at time of transfer. Post-procedure notes include the patient's condition on arrival back to the unit or at the completion of the procedure, use of any equipment or tubes, education, family present, procedures or treatments started, and appropriate monitoring per orders or standards.

Refusal of Treatment

If a patient refuses treatment, the refusal must be documented. You should clearly document what the patient is refusing and why, your efforts to educate the patient about the need for the treatment, risks of not having treatment, your communication of the situation to the doctor and supervisor, and the fact that treatment was not provided because of the patient's refusal. The patient has every right to refuse any treatment. If you require the legally competent patient to undergo a treatment (s)he has refused, you could be charged with assault and battery. Your job is to give the patient enough information to make an informed decision. If the patient is reluctant to take the treatment even after receiving education, inform the doctor so that (s)he can talk with the patient. It is extremely important to document any refusals of treatment to protect yourself, the agency, and the doctor. If the patient's refusal leads to complications, your documentation will be useful if there are any legal repercussions. If your facility has a Refusal of Treatment Release form, ask the patient to sign it. If the patient refuses to sign the release form, note that fact in the record.

Adverse Reactions

Document all adverse reactions to any treatments and continue documenting until the problem is resolved. An adverse reaction can be anything from a tape burn to cardiac arrest. You need to document the reaction, when you identified the reaction, the extent of the reaction, report of reaction to doctor, patient education, treatment, monitoring, and the response to treatment.

Patient Injury

Patient injuries include more than adverse reactions. Falls, surgical injuries, equipment-induced injuries, and self-induced injuries are all types of patient injuries. You should document the patient's account of the injury in the patient's own words, what you observed, witnesses, what the witnesses observed, extent of injury, to whom you reported the injury (supervisor and doctor), patient education, treatment, and monitoring. You will need to make an incident or occurrence report. DO NOT document that you wrote a report in the patient's record.

Codes: Cardiac, Respiratory, or Complete

If the patient goes into cardiac, respiratory, or complete arrest, you must document the code. As people arrive on the scene, one nurse should be assigned the responsibility of documenting what happens during the code. Most facilities document codes on flow sheets, but you will usually need to make a narrative note to supplement the flow sheet. You need to document, either on the flow sheet or on the narrative note, everything that happened before, during, and after the code. Your narrative note should start with a short history of the event and other important information such as times of events, personnel present, medications, treatments, response to medication or treatments, any notifications, and postcode care or disposition. Be sure to document that CPR was started promptly, if that is the case.

Telephone Calls

Communication with doctors, outside agencies, clergy, and family should be documented fully in the patient's record. Sometimes you will need to document communication with other departments in your institution, such as when performing or requesting a consultation. You need to document when you made the call, who was called, what you told the person, the results of the call, and treatments initiated after the call.

It is extremely important that you keep the patient's doctor advised of any patient problems or changes. You need to document these problems or changes, but you must also notify the physician in a timely manner. This usually means telephoning the doctor. As noted above, you must document any communication you have with the doctor in the patient's behalf. You should call the doctor about any changes in the patient's condition or any of the following situations:

- Unusual occurrence
- Accidents/falls
- Abnormal test results
- Errors in medications
- Inability to carry out physician's orders
- Questions about any order
- Residents failing to take appropriate action
- Usual monitoring test not being ordered (to verify that the monitoring test was not accidentally missed)
- Family concerns and questions
- Information that would affect discharge planning[2]

Occurrence of Error

You must document an error. For example, if you give the patient the wrong medication, you must document that fact nonjudgmentally. State that you gave medication X, dosage, monitoring of patient, to whom the incident was reported (supervisor and doctor), what you told them, and treatments/monitoring started. Do not make an apology or incriminate yourself: just state the facts.

An incident or occurrence report must be written. DO NOT document that you wrote an incident report in the record.

Unscheduled Medications

Doctors will often order several types of prn medications. These orders often include medication for pain, nausea, and constipation. If you give the medication, the administration is documented in the Medication Administration Record (MAR) and followed up with documentation stating why the prn medication was required. Document any other unscheduled medications such as a single-dose medication ordered by the doctor. Single-dose medications could include a supplemental dose of furosemide (Lasix) or digoxin (Lanoxin).

Documentation should address that you gave the medication, why you give it, dose, route, time, and results. If you gave pain medication, did the patient get relief? If you gave a dose of Lasix what was the urinary output, blood pressure, and lung sounds? Did the problem resolve after the medication was administered? If not what did you do? You want to document clearly that the physician's orders were followed and completed, and if not, why not. If you do not follow an order, you need to document why, who was informed, and the response to that contact.

Spiritual Interventions

You should document any baptisms, last rites, or any other religious ceremonies. Remember, we treat the whole patient, both religious and physiologic needs. Because the clergy usually do not have documentation privileges, you are responsible for documentation.

Living Will Declarations

The federal Patient Self-Determination Act of 1990 [42 U.S.C. Section 1395(a)(1)(Q)] requires federally funded institutions to advise patients of their right to accept or refuse medical treatment. The goal of the Act is to inform the patient of his/her right to make health care decisions while still competent. Most states have their own laws regarding living wills and durable power of attorney. You need to know the laws in your state. The Act states that on admission the patient must be told and given written material regarding living wills and durable power of attorney for health care. Many institutions give the main responsibility of meeting the Patient Self-Determination Act to non-nursing staff, but you may be given those responsibilities. You should document any interactions you have with a patient and/or his family regarding the Act, including patient education and patient's response. You should also document notification of doctor. A copy of the documents should be filed in the patient's chart. If the patient has a living will or durable power of attorney, but did not bring it, have the family bring it in as soon as possible. If the patient makes any changes to these legal instruments, you should again document the changes and advise the doctor.[3]

Unexpected Events

Any unusual change in the patient's condition or unusual event in the patient's life that affects the ability for self-care must be documented. For example, an elderly patient with a hip fracture is expected to go home with his daughter until he can care for himself and return to his home. Yesterday, his daughter experienced a heart attack, which invalidated that plan. You need to document that his caretaker is no longer available as well as your plans to help the patient address the issue. These plans would include any consult initiated or discussions with other family members.

Transfer

When a patient is transferred from your unit to another unit or facility, you must summarize the patient's stay up to the point of transfer. This summary will show the patient's condition on transfer. A copy is sent to the receiving agency or is available for patients transferred within the facility. The information gives the receiving unit sufficient information to care appropriately for the patient. The transfer note is very similar to an admission note. It should be brief and include patient history, current condition, reason for transfer, nursing diagnoses, results of care, and patient teaching completed and uncompleted. Also included are age, sex, vital signs, mode of transfer, notification of family, allergies, medication records, and disposition of valuables.

If a patient is transferred within your facility, the records are also transferred to the next unit. In this case, the note may not need to be as extensive, but you need to ensure that the information is available to the new staff. Be extremely careful to provide an adequate, current picture of the patient's condition on transfer.

For patients being transferred to another facility, it is important to be complete when writing your transfer note. In this situation, you will essentially write a discharge note along with the transfer note. Most facilities have a transfer summary that addresses most of the preceding issues. If yours does not, be sure to supplement the form with adequate narrative documentation. For those patients going to a nursing home, you may need to assist in completing forms designed by the state, the receiving facility, or both to ensure that the receiving facility can give the appropriate level of care.

To document compliance with COBRA regulations, the following information should be included:

- Patient or surrogate refuses consent to examination or treatment, refuses consent to an appropriate transfer, or requests transfer to another facility.
- A responsible physician certifies that the medical benefits of transfer outweigh the risks of not transferring the patient and that the transfer is done correctly.
- That the patient was informed of the risks and benefits of the plan of care.
- Informed consent from the patient refusing treatment.
- That the patient was informed of the benefits and risks of the transfer.[4]

Your underlying goals in all documentation situations are to ensure quality patient care and to legally protect, yourself, the doctor, and the facility.

Discharge

At discharge the main events of the patient's hospitalization should be summarized in a discharge nursing note. This note should describe the patient's current condition and ability to do self-care and should indicate that appropriate post-hospital care was planned for and is available. Future care requirements must be clearly delineated, with appropriate documentation as to how those needs will be met.

When writing a discharge summary, the following information should be addressed: summary of care, current status regarding each nursing diagnosis treated during hospitalization, unusual events or findings, inpatient teaching, where patient is discharged to, in care of whom (by name), discharge address, mode of transportation home (car, taxi, bus, or medical transport), discharge teaching, name of any agencies involved with post-hospitalization care, patient's ability to perform self-care, what needs to be done after hospitalization, and who will do the care or teaching. Discharge teaching should include diagnosis, diet, medications, activity level, special care, follow-up, referrals, and patient's understanding of the same.

Most hospitals have preprinted discharge summary and instruction sheets that you must complete. Your responsibility is to ensure that you document the information outlined above and within the format required by the institution.

Techniques of Documentation

When writing a nursing note, the following guidelines must be followed to maintain standards of documentation and to develop a legally sound record.

- Use correct chart.
- Use correct form.
- Fill out forms completely and correctly.
- Ensure proper identification on form. Each form should be imprinted with the patient's information card. At a minimum, each form should contain the patient's name and identification number.
- Use black ink, blue only if approved by your facility.
- Use the first available line on progress notes to make your entry.
- Start each note with a date (including month, day, and year) and time (use either military or standard time as approved by your facility).
- Use actual time entry made for date/time entry and indicate time of events in the body of the note.
- Organize your thoughts before writing a note. Group together all information that relates to the same problem; this is especially important when writing notes using the narrative note format.

- Avoid repeating information by referring reader to previous entries or other documentation forms.
- Make yourself or other team members the implied subject of the sentence For example, "walked patient" instead "patient walked."
- Write neatly and legibly.
- Use complete sentences or phrases that convey meaning clearly.
- Use brief, clear, and concise statements of the facts.
- Use correct grammar.
- Use correct spelling. Carry a small notebook with words you often have trouble spelling, (I have successfully used a small pocket address book.) **Use the dictionary!**
- Use facility-approved abbreviations; just because an abbreviation is used in one facility does not mean that it is approved in all facilities. Use abbreviations carefully. Make sure your meaning is clear and understandable now and in the unspecific future.
- Use appropriate terminology. Be sure you know how to use the term correctly. You do not need to impress anyone by using fancy terms; keep it simple.
- Be sure you know the exact meaning of medical terms before using them.
- The use of "I" is permissible.
- Use measurable terms. State "walked 30 feet with assistance of walker, escorted by one staff member." Not "walked in hall."
- Use centimeters or millimeters to record measurements. Do not record measurements by comparing what you are measuring to pieces of fruit, vegetables, or other nonspecific objects.
- Be specific. Do not be tentative. Choose your terms carefully.

- Clearly identify care that was given by others, especially those who are not permitted to document.
- Document your own care; document for those who can document only if you have firsthand knowledge of the event or care.
- Use the patient's terms to describe subjective symptoms.
- If you paraphrase a patient's comments, be sure that you do not change the meaning of the comments. Paraphrase using brief, accurate statements.
- Use patient and family quotes when exact words are necessary to convey strong meanings or when paraphrasing would alter the meaning.
- End each note with your signature, including credentials (RN or LPN).
- Always place a whole number or zero in front of a decimal point, for example "0.125" not ".125." You can kill a patient by the misplacement of a decimal.
- Line out any unused space at the end of a note.
- Line out spaces on forms that do not apply to a particular patient or mark N/A (if approved by your facility) in the space.
- Notes by student nurses may need to be co-signed by an RN, check your hospital policies and procedures.
- If it is necessary to recopy a page, mark the recopied page as recopied. Save both copies in the chart. Mark the top of the recopied page with "Notes recopied from the original 3 Jan 93." If you copy your own notes, at the same time the original note was written and they are the only notes on the page, the original note does not need to be saved.

- Terms used in the nursing progress notes should correspond to those terms used in the care plan and doctor's orders.
- Use the facility-approved method to correct mistakes. Draw a single line through the incorrect entry. Mark over the entry with either "error," "delete," or "mistaken entry" (whichever is approved), your initials, and date.
- Clearly identify late entries. Never ask someone to leave you space to document information. Go to the next available line and note date and time you are making the entry. Follow with the words "Late Entry," date and time of the event you are documenting; why the note was late; and the information that needs to be documented.
- Follow your facility's documentation policies and procedures.

What to Document

Information noted below will be documented in one of several different areas in a patient's medical record. You will use nursing (patient) progress notes, flow sheets, medication administration records, and graphic sheets to document patient care and status. Hospital guidelines and nursing policies and procedures will determine where you document pertinent patient data. You should document the following information:

- Nursing concerns whether they are called focus, diagnosis, or problem.
- Patient status.
- Implementation of doctor or other health care team members orders, including procedures and diagnostic tests.
- Interventions in response to a patient problem, always documented after completion, never before.

- Assessment and reassessment of the patient and his/her problems, including negative as well as positive findings.
- Amount of time required to perform procedures and reason that more than the usual amount of time is needed, if necessary.
- Amount of supplies used and the number of staff required to complete the task.
- Patient's and/or family's limitations and ability to perform the care; what you did to overcome any shortcomings.
- Patient and family education, instructions, and counseling.
- Signs and symptoms, including psychosocial.
- Abilities or inabilities to perform activities of daily living.
- Communication problems with the patient and/or family.
- The fact that and reasons why patient and/or family refuses treatments, medications, or procedures. Include your interventions, education, and notifications in the event of a refusal.
- Time, route, dosage, and site of medications.
- All monitoring activities.
- Response to care, interventions, and/or treatments; evidence that patient is meeting the nursing care plan expected outcomes.
- Revisions of the care plan or education plan and the reasons for the revisions.
- Professional judgments, preceded by information on which judgment is based.
- Comfort, safety, and surveillance activities, such as bed rails up, call light within reach, or constant supervision in playroom.
- Patient's possession of any unauthorized items including home medications, smoking materials (if the hospital has no smoking policies), personal electrical equipment

(not approved by the medical repair department), and alcohol.

- Any incidents both in the record and on the incident or occurrence report; do not place blame, just report the facts.
- All observations regarding the patient, including patient interactions with family or significant others, especially those interactions that help explain current problems and support mechanisms.
- That informed consent was obtained.
- Patient's compliance and noncompliance with medical and nursing instructions.
- Any patient or family actions that could potentially contribute or cause injury or possibly death. Examples could include the removal of traction, smoking in bed, refusal of treatments, failure to follow safety instructions, and tampering with hospital equipment.
- Any patient or family comments about bringing lawsuits against your facility or any other facility. Remember to report these comments to your supervisor.
- Any information reported to the doctor and the response. Be very specific about noting the time you communicated with doctor and the information conveyed to the doctor. Indicate that you called the doctor. Use "Notified Dr. X" not "Dr. X called." The latter leaves ambiguous the question of who called whom. Finish the note by documenting the doctor's response.
- Information from flow sheets that you need to elaborate about.
- Assessment information not documented on flow sheet.
- Use of equipment and patient's response to the equipment.

- The results of multidisciplinary care conferences.
- Use of any unusual amount of supplies and the reasons why for supplies that are charged to the patient. If the insurance auditors cannot determine a reason for the amount of supplies used, they will not pay for them.
- Reasons why any treatment was withheld or modified.
- Attempts to reach the doctor and your actions when you could not reach him/her in a reasonable amount of time. Follow the facility's policies and procedures to ensure that the patient's problem is dealt with expeditiously.
- Patient's refusal or inability to give medical history and information regarding the current problem, medications, and treatments. If the patient is medically unable to respond, document your attempts to get the information from other sources.
- Information regarding the Patient Self-Determination Act.
- Describe jewelry by color and appearance, not by the type of metal or gem.

Documentation Enhancements

You can enhance your documentation by some of the following practices:

- Chart promptly after the event when possible.
- Take frequent notes if you will not be documenting immediately.
- Use the nursing process to organize your thoughts as you write a note. Think assessment, nursing diagnosis, expected outcomes, planning, intervention, and evaluation as you write your notes.
- Know and meet your facility's standards of documentation.

71

- Read previous nursing and medical progress notes. Followup earlier notes with appropriate patient observations.
- Use previous notes and records to jog your memory about information that needs to be documented.
- Use drawings or sketches to illustrate what you are trying to describe.
- As you document, address current problems. Review resolved problems. Are they still inactive? You should document reassessment at a reasonable interval. Ask yourself, does the patient have physical, emotional, spiritual, or social needs that I have not addressed? What have I done for this patient? What orders have I carried out today? With whom have I communicated about this patient? What have I learned today about this patient?
- Follow any patient report of subjective symptoms with objective information when possible, as well as your nursing actions.

To optimize the use of the patient's record, make documenting a priority, be thorough in your documentation, and keep it current.

Pitfalls of Documentation

Records that do not clearly show that the nurses and facility are meeting the basic standards of care acceptable for the nursing area can cause you to lose any lawsuit brought against you or the facility. That is why you need to follow the documentation guidelines outlined earlier. You also need to avoid several pitfalls that can decrease your record's viability in a court of law.

DO NOT:

- Fail to follow documentation guidelines.
- Fail to comply with facility policy and procedures regarding care to be rendered.
- Use ditto marks.

- Document for someone else unless absolutely necessary. If necessary clearly identify who did the task.
- Sign anyone else's nurses notes.
- Leave blank lines or spaces in documentation or on forms.
- Chart before the event, such as giving medications. What happens if a patient refuses a medication you have signed off? How would you explain to a court of law why you deleted the 7PM note saying that the patient was resting comfortably and followed it with a note of a serious deteriorating of the patient's condition.
- Express opinions or assumptions.
- Criticize or blame other team members.
- Tamper with a record including any official logs kept on the unit.
- Use correcting fluid, tape, or erasures to correct errors.
- Back date records.
- Lie or misrepresent information.
- Try to prejudice the reader.
- Insert information between lines.
- Use erasable ink.
- Document that an incident or occurrence report was filed.
- Fail to document communication with doctors and the content of that communication.
- Use unmeasurable or vague terms such as *good*, *better*, *negative*, *appears*, and *seems*.
- Fail to document incidents.
- Add information to a chart that will be used in a lawsuit.
- Allow *anyone* to pressure you from documenting the facts by adding or withholding information. Report anyone who applies pressure to your supervisor. If your supervisor is pressuring you, go to the next person in

the chain of authority, the risk management director, or the hospital lawyer.

- Discard part or all of a medical record.
- Alter anyone else's notes or documentation. Report to your supervisor any evidence that a chart or notation has been altered.
- Document in a biased or negative manner. Do not demean the patient with words such as *useless*, *lazy*, *bum*, *drunk*, or *disagreeable*. Chart the facts.
- Use unapproved abbreviations or shorthand notations when documenting. Write out words. For example, do not use T3 or Tyl 3 for Tylenol #3.
- List account numbers from credit cards when inventorying valuables.

Some abbreviations and apothecary symbols should not be used because they can be misinterpreted, leading to critical errors. Do not use the apothecary symbols for ounce, dram, or minim. Write out the term unit. Do not use *u*. It can be misread as a zero when poorly written.

Remember: One of your goals when documenting is to provide an accurate report of the patient's care, health status, and stay in your facility. Information must be complete, unbiased, legible, and understandable today and in the unspecified future.

Although the main purpose of strong documentation is to provide quality patient care, you must also be aware of your legal responsibilities. If you cannot read or understand your note or abbreviations while you are on the courtroom stand, how will the jury assess your credibility? When reviewing a record before testifying in court, you must not alter the record to coverup previous inadequate documentation, care deficiencies, or facts that demonstrate negligence.

One of your goals when documenting is to provide an accurate report of the patient's care, health status, and stay in your facility. Information must be complete, unbiased, legible, and understandable today and in the unspecified future.

Any information you find or document in a patient's medical record is confidential. Any release of that information to anyone that does not have the legal right or need to know that information is a breach of the patient's confidentially. This breach is a criminal offense. Remember the statement: "What you see or hear here stays here."

Summary

This chapter has emphasized the following key points:

1. Nurses must document to meet their professional responsibilities at very specific times including

> admission
> changes or lack of in patient's
>   condition
> new nursing diagnosis
> problems resolved
> pre-procedure/post-procedure
> refusal of treatment
> adverse reactions
> patient injury
> codes
> telephone calls
> occurrence of error
> unscheduled medications
> spiritual interventions
> living will declarations
> unexpected events
> transfers
> discharge

2. Follow guidelines when writing a nursing note to make the note the most meaningful for the patient and to protect yourself legally.
3. Documented information should be patient-centered.
4. When documenting, information may be added or deleted, that can decrease the legal importance of the record and cause you to lose any legal action brought against you.

This chapter contains much important information. You are encouraged to reread it before continuing to read the manual.

References

1. Fischback, F. T. (1991). *Documenting Care Communication, the Nursing Process and Documentation Standard*. Philadelphia: F. A. Davis Co., 272–278.
2. Dill-Calloway, S. (1993). *The Law for Nurses Who Supervise and Manage Others*. Eau Claire, WI: Professional Education Systems, 256.
3. Greve, Paul. (1991). Legally Speaking: Advance Directives—What the New Law Means to You. *RN*, *54*(11), 63–64.
4. Dill-Calloway, S. (1993). *The Law for Nurses Who Supervise and Manage Others*. Eau Claire, WI: Professional Education Systems, Inc., 265–266.

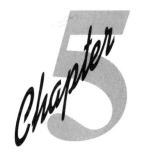

Writing Summary and Evaluative Nursing Notes

Chapter 5

Objectives

The learner will be able to:
1. Write complete, concise, and clear nursing notes including
   A. Summaries: admission, transfers, discharge, and death
   B. Evaluative statements
2. Write admission, transfer, discharge, and evaluative notes that reflect the patient's response to nursing care.

You have seen when and what you should document. Now we will explore the how of writing nursing notes. You will write three types of nursing notes: summary notes, evaluative statements, and progress notes. Your notes must inform the reader about the patient so that the health care team can give quality patient care efficiently and economically. This chapter discusses summary notes and evaluative statements. Chapter 6 discusses progress notes.

Summary Notes

The nurse uses summary notes to organize a large volume of data in order to communicate patient status and needs, communicate between nursing units or facilities, and identify patient concerns during the covered time. You will routinely be writing four types of summaries: admissions, transfer, discharge, and death. In other situations, you may be required to write summaries of a patient's care and health status that cover a specific time period, such as weekly, bi-weekly, or monthly. A correctly written summary must be organized and succinct because it is vital for continuity of care at very specific times in a patient's hospitalization. Summary notes are long and take time to organize appropriately, so plan your time accordingly.

Admission Notes

The admission note is the first narrative note you write about a patient. It organizes information obtained from the nursing admission assessment, physical examination, and clinical data and any other data you have about the patient into a synopsis of the patient's current health status.

While writing the admission note you want to:

- Show justification for hospitalization
- Establish patient's condition on arrival
- Identify nursing needs
- Document the use of the nursing process
- Establish goals for care

As you prepare to write, remember that the patient is a person with his/her own past, present, and future. He or she has hopes, dreams, and fears and is part of a family, job, and community. The patient is not a "pre-op gallbladder" or "the MI in room 611B."

Let's look at an admission note, Example 5-1, that you could write for Mrs. Wilbur who was admitted with a diagnosis of pneumonia.

Example 5-1: Admission–Medical

Date/Time	Focus	Progress Note
17 Jan 93 1830	Admission assessment	DATA: 67 y/o female Caucasian housewife admitted to room 611B, at 1745, by wheelchair from admissions accompanied by admitting clerk and husband. Diagnosis LLL pneumonia under care of Dr. Gray, Internal Medicine. No known allergies. Complains of severe cough for 3 days, today developed a productive cough, green sputum. Produces about a tablespoon of sputum each morning. Fever intermittently for 2 days, 103.5°F maximum, relieved by ASA. Has pain in L lower chest with deep inspiration and coughing. Pain 4 (scale 1–10, 10 severe). Often awakened by coughing. Denies chills or dyspnea. Lungs clear, except crackles LLL, on auscultation. BP 138/82 T 103.2°F P 102 R 28. States tires easily. Lips and mucous membranes dry. Urine dark amber. O_2 sat 88% on room air. Treatment before seeing Dr. Gray this AM was ASA and cough drops. Patient gave husband wallet & jewelry to take home. History of MI '89 and CHF '90.————
	Fluid volume deficit R/T fever	
	Pain R/T frequent coughing and inflammation	
	High risk for impaired gas exchange	
		ACTION: Called Dr. Gray at 1810 and notified him of arrival and temperature, see additional orders. IV started, see IV flow sheet. O_2 on 2 L per nasal cannula. HOB in semi-Fowler's. Admission labs including blood cultures drawn by lab tech, at 1813. UA and C & S specimen sent to lab at 1815. Antibiotic therapy then started and Tylenol given, see MAR. Demonstrated cough and deep breathing, use of incentive spirometer, splinting, maintaining intake and output, as well as ——————(Continued) *F. Honn RN*

79

(Continued) 17 Jan 93 1830		explained importance of each. Instructed to cough and deep breathe, use spirometer, turn, and drink glass of H_2O or juice q1h while awake and q2h at night. Patient able to return demonstrations appropriately. See care plan for specific plan of care. Plan of care reviewed with patient & husband and they concur with plan. Will recheck temperature at 1915. Personal items placed close, call light within reach, and side rails up. Patient instructed to call for help when getting up.———————————————— RESPONSE: Patient lying quietly in bed dozing, husband at bedside. O_2 saturation 94% at 1815 on 2 L of O_2.—— *F. Honn RN*
17 Jan 93 1920	Fluid Volume deficit	RESPONSE: T 101.8°F, drinking fluids well, 450cc since admission. *F. Honn RN*

Compare the preceding note with a more complex situation.

Example 5-2:
Admission–Orthopedic

Date/Time	Focus	Progress Note

15 May 92
1115
	Admission
	   assessment
	
	Pain R hip
	Safety
	Circulatory Status
	   R leg
		DATA: 105 y/o retired Native American male admitted at 1015 via stretcher to Rm 213B from ER, accompanied by Dr. Brown and Mrs. Keller RN. Diagnosis fractured R. Hip after falling out of bed this AM at the nursing home. Under care of Dr. Brown Orthopedic Services. R hip with obvious deformity, large hard lump. Patient uses L foot attempting to move R leg past the midline. Circ check of feet shows: capillary refill <3 seconds, feet warm and pink, no edema, moans every time touched. Speaks only Navajo. Mrs. Yazzie, interpreter, states patient unable to answer questions coherently, is
		———— (Continued) *D. Wilson RN*

(Continued) 15 May 92
1115

chanting. BP 170/96 T 98.7°F P 100 R 18. All skin intact with 2 cm by 3 cm bruise on R shoulder.————————————
ACTION: Eggcrate on bed. Placed in 10 pounds Bucks traction, R leg. Bed alarm on. Medicated for pain, see MAR. IV started, see IV flow sheet. Will move closer to nurse's station as soon as possible. Will call nursing home to get a patient history, including allergies to complete nursing assessment. Consult sent to discharge planner to assure that present nursing home will be able to care for patient post-op and because of patient's age. See plan of care.————
RESPONSE: Chanting decreased after traction applied and medicated.————
—————————————D. Wilson RN

The first few sentences of the admission note describes the patient. Age, sex, ethnic background, and occupation provides a better understanding of the patient's life experiences and the possibility of coping with the illness. This information allows you to sort out problems or illnesses related to that background and heritage. It will also give you ideas about how to approach patient education. You must remember that how you approach patient teaching depends not only on education levels but also on coping skills, emotional status, stress levels, support systems, and prior experiences.

The admission assessment summary provides direction for future nursing care after you make the nursing diagnosis which is based on the existing information. For example, the patient with pneumonia requires nursing care to reduce the temperature, improve hydration, and decrease pain. The direction of care will change as the patient's condition changes or new information becomes available leading to other health care problems.

Exercise 5-1

Do these two examples of admission notes meet the guideline for writing admission summaries? To find out, reexamine the two notes and answer the following questions.

1. Why is the patient in the hospital?

   67-year-old woman   105-year-old man

   _____   _____

   _____   _____

2. If given the following information in a later progress note, can you tell whether the patient is improving? Circle the appropriate answer.

   C/O difficulty breathing.   Demerol at 1200, asleep at 1230.

   Improving/Deteriorating   Improving/Deteriorating

3. Nursing needs arise out of patient problems. Do you agree with the nursing focus? Circle your answer.

   Yes/No   Yes/No

4. What statements in the note would you associate with each component of the nursing process?

   Assessment

   _____   _____

   _____   _____

   Nursing Diagnosis

   _____   _____

   _____   _____

   Expected Outcomes

   _____   _____

   _____   _____

67-year-old woman   105-year-old man

Planning

————————————————   ————————————————
————————————————   ————————————————

Intervention

————————————————   ————————————————
————————————————   ————————————————

Evaluation

————————————————   ————————————————
————————————————   ————————————————

5. What statements tell you the plan of care?

————————————————   ————————————————
————————————————   ————————————————

6. Were the objectives met?
   Yes/No   Yes/No

Your charting skills will grow as you gain more charting experience. Keep practicing and reviewing other charting, remembering to use the guidelines.

Transfer Notes

Transfer notes should be written when you transfer a patient between units of the hospital and between facilities. The goal of transfer notes is to provide the receiving unit with sufficient information to guarantee continuity of care. Transfers can happen as a patient improves or deteriorates or requires care that is unavailable on your unit or in your facility.

To illustrate a typical transfer note, let's return to Mrs. Wilbur. Two days after she was admitted to the hospital with pneumonia, Mrs. Wilbur had a heart attack and had to be transferred to the CCU. Your note may look like the following example.

Example 5-3: Transfer Between Hospital Units

Focus	Progress Note
Transfer Summary	DATA: 67 y/o female Caucasian housewife admitted on 17 Jan with diagnosis of LLL pneumonia. Has been treated for: 1) Fluid volume deficit R/T fever. Treated with IV fluids and oral hydration. I & O now equal, last 24 I=2400 & O=2300, urine sp gr 1.010 and color light straw yellow, mucous membrane moist. Fever treated with antibiotic therapy & tylenol. Fever range in last 24 hours 99.8 - 100.5°F. 2) Pain R/T frequent coughing and inflammation. Pain has been controlled with Tylenol #3 with decreased use of pain med in last 24 hours. Cough decreasing to coughing spells when arises or becomes active, no longer keeps awake at night. 3) High risk for impaired gas exchange R/T infection. Uses O_2 after activity and at night, but pulls off after lying quietly in bed for 15 minutes. O_2 sat on room air when lying in bed is 92%. Being transferred to CCU to R/O myocardial infarct. Developed sudden severe substernal chest pain radiation to L jaw. Skin dusky, warm, and diaphoretic. Dyspneic. EKG shows ST elevation, T inverted, with widening QRS, and multiple PVCs. Treated with O_2, sublingual nitroglycerine I/150 gr X 3 (no relief), 10mg IV morphine. Monitor shows frequent PVCs. O_2 3 L/ nasal cannula. O_2 sat 96%. Placed in high Fowler's position. BP 102/68 down from average of 130s/80s, T 99.8°F P 93 R 26. At time of transfer pain is resolved, skin cool and damp, dyspnea decrease by 50%, and BP 110/76 P 88 R 22. Allergies: NKDA. Valuables were sent home on admission.———————— ACTION: Dr. Gray will call husband. Supervisor, Mrs. Jefferson, notified of patient's condition and now on unit. Called report to Mrs. Taylor, RN in CCU then transferred by bed, with O_2 at 3 L/nasal cannula, and on portable monitor. Accompanied by Dr. Gray, myself, and supervisor. ———————— RESPONSE: Patient arrived in CCU unchanged from earlier assessment. ———————————— *S. Estever RN*

Because the patient was transferred within the same facility, the note could have been shorter. The critical element is the documentation of what occurred just before the transfer.

Another example of a transfer note describes the transfer of the patient with the fractured hip back to the nursing home.

Example 5-4: Transfer and Discharge to a Nursing Home

Focus	Progress Note
Transfer & Discharge Summary	DATA: 105 y/o Native American male admitted on 15 May after fracturing R hip after falling out of bed. Had surgery 16 May for compression screw placement. Nursing problems include: 1) Pain: initially required Demerol 75mg, but gets good relief with Tylenol #3 two tabs 2 or 3 times a day. 2) Circulatory status R leg: circulation checks good through hospitalization: capillary refill <3 sec, feet warm and pink, able to feel light sensation, and no distal edema. Swelling of R hip developed post-op, but now 90% resolved. Remains confused unable to assess for numbness or tingling. 3) Safety: Remains confused and chants when tired or in pain. Able to feed self. Needs total help with hygiene and elimination. Needs safety belt when up in chair because he tends to slip towards front of chair. Needs side rails when in bed. 4) Mobility: had b.i.d. PT treatments and now able to transfer with help of one, which was the limit of ambulation before injury. Incision clean and dry, no redness or drainage, Steri-Strips in place. Family notified of today's transfer, by Mrs. Bekan, RN Discharge Planner. Allergic to PENICILLIN. Came to ward without valuables. BP 126/86 T 98.8°F P 88 R 18. On digoxin 0.125mg q.d., Colace 100mg b.i.d. Tylenol #3 one or two tablets q4h prn. Transferred to Rest Manor Nursing Home for long-term nursing care.——————— ACTION: Report called to Mrs. Clark RN, staff nurse at Rest Manor Nursing Home. Transferred via gurney by City EMS, transfer records given to EMS attendants.—— *P. Pizzuto LPN*

Discharge Notes

Discharge notes are written to summarize nursing care given during hospitalization and to establish the patient's status on discharge. The nursing discharge summary complements the doctor's discharge summary. The doctor discuss the pathology of the illness; the nurse summarizes the patient's response to the pathology.

After a stay in the CCU, Mrs. Wilbur was transferred back to your unit and is now ready for discharge.

Example 5-5: Discharge–Medical

Date/Time	Focus	Progress Note
26 Jan 93	Discharge	DATA: 67 y/o female housewife admitted
0910	Summary	with LLL pneumonia 17 Jan 93 and had
		an uncomplicated inferior wall MI on 19
		Jan. Admission vitals BP 138/82 T 103.2°F
		P 102 R 28. Nursing Diagnosis addressed
		includes: 1) Fluid Volume Deficit R/T
		Fever, resolved. Afebrile since 21 Jan,
		temperature now 99°F or less. Intake
		and Output balanced, mucous membranes
		moist, urine clear yellow, and urine sp gr
		on 23 Jan 1.015. 2) Pain R/T frequent
		coughing, inflammation, and myocardial
		ischemia resolved. Denies all pain and
		cough. Last pain medication was 24 Jan.
		for any type of pain. Last cardiac pain 21
		Jan. 3) High risk for impaired gas
		exchange R/T infection, resolved.
		Ambulates and does self-care without
		dyspnea, diaphoresis, and easily tiring.
		No edema of feet and hands. Lungs clear
		bilaterally on auscultation. 4) Anxiety
		R/T Uncertainty of Physical Condition.
		States she is no longer scared like she was
		the first two nights in CCU. Has been re-
		laxed in appearance since return to unit.
		States she and her husband have been
		through this before and they did okay and
		they will be again. Reports husband
		very supportive, as are children, he is quick
		to do household chores. Discharge vital
		signs at 0600 this AM BP 136/84 T 99.8°F
		P 80 R 20 Has gone through Cardiac
		Didactic Education program, see form
		2034. Completed inpatient Cardiac Rehab
		program without difficulty, see form
		2035. Wants to lose 5 more pounds, was
		seen by dietitian and will be followed by
		Cardiac Rehab dietitian as an outpatient.
		ACTION: Discharge instructions ————
		————(Continued) *K. Baird RN*

| (Continued) | 26 Jan 93 0910 | reviewed with patient, see Discharge Instruction Summary. Discharge to care of Daniel Wilbur, husband. Will be returning to own home locally. Taken by wheelchair to lobby and left in privately owned vehicle.——————————— RESPONSE: Able to repeat instructions and verbalizes intent to follow through with appointments and Cardiac Rehab. Clearly states what medications on, use, dosage, frequency, and side effects. —— —————————————————— *K. Baird RN* |

The following example is a discharge note for a surgical patient.

Example 5-6: Discharge–Surgical

| Focus Discharge Summary | Progress Note DATA: 43 y/o Black female accountant admitted 20 Jan 93 with diagnosis of endometriosis. Admission vital signs BP 128/82 T 98.5°F P 74 R 12. Total Abdominal Hysterectomy and Bilateral Salpingo-Oophorectomy performed under general anesthesia on 21 Jan. Nursing diagnoses resolved or no longer at risk for include: 1) High Risk For Infection R/T abdominal incision and indwelling catheter. Afebrile for last 48 hours. Had 99.8 - 100.8°F temp intermittently for first 24 hours, which was successfully treated with po fluids, incentive spirometer, and deep breathing exercises. Suture line clean, dry and edges well approximated. No redness, drainage, or foul odor. Steri-Strips intact. 2) Altered Patterns of Urinary Elimination R/T Indwelling Catheter. Catheter removed at 0600 on 22 Jan. Voided 6 hours later for 300cc, no difficulty voiding thereafter. 3) Pain R/T abdominal surgery. Pain controlled with po Tylenol #3. Ambulatory and able to do self-care with minimal assistance. 4) Body Image Disturbance R/T Actual Loss of Reproductive Capability. States she and husband are happy with three children and did not want any more. Had concerns before surgery, but feels has made right decision. Vital signs 0600 today BP 126/78 T 98.7°F P 72 R 14. ACTION: Discharge instructions reviewed with patient, see —————————————————————— (Continued) *G. Bass RN* |

| (Continued) | Discharge Instructions Summary. Discharged to her home locally, address on face sheet verified, in care of Herbert Wilson, husband. To lobby by wheelchair and left in taxi.——————————— RESPONSE: Patient explained proper medication administration routine, how to care for wound, lists signs and symptoms of infection to watch for, when to see doctor, and what to do if problem develops. Expresses intent on keeping scheduled appointments.——————————————— *G. Bass RN* |

Death Summaries

A summary about a patient who has expired is essentially the same as a discharge note with a few additional facts. A death summary should include time life signs ceased, time a doctor notified, time patient's doctor notified (if not the same doctor that was called to assist with emergency situation), time death pronounced and by whom, which family members present, time family notified if not present at the death, and disposition of body and valuables.

Evaluative Statements

As a nurse, you have a professional responsibility and obligation to evaluate your patient. You document your findings as an evaluative statement in the nursing progress notes. A properly written evaluative statement consists of two components:

- The data on which your judgments are based
- Your professional judgment.

Evaluative statements are based on objective information, which is information you have obtained through physical assessment, observation, monitoring, laboratory data, or data supplied by someone other than the patient. Objective information is measurable and verifiable. An evaluative statement is based on objective data, but can and should be supported with subjective data.

Evaluative statements are used in the following situations:

- Assessment: You show that the problem is amenable to nursing intervention leading to a nursing diagnosis.
- Reassessment: Defining the patient's current status regarding a nursing diagnosis. The goal of reassessment is to find any indication of the patient's response or lack of response to medical and nursing interventions.
- Discharge: Each nursing diagnosis is reviewed, and the patient's current status is compared to the expected outcome for that diagnosis. Then an evaluation is made to see if the problem is resolved or the patient is no longer at risk. If the patient is still at risk or the problem is not resolved, you indicate how the problem will be addressed at home.

You have already seen evaluation and evaluative statements in admission and discharge assessments. Now we will look at the documentation of reassessment evaluations.

Evaluative statements are made during the course of the hospitalization to help guide and direct individualized care. You are always making evaluations of the patient's progress. You often make a judgment unconsciously, which then leads to further patient evaluation. You may hear an offhand comment, see a look, or just get an undefined gut feeling about a patient. Those comments, looks, or feelings may not be scientific; but based on experience, you know that further information has to be collected. The result of that assessment often leads to an evaluative statement. Your findings are then the basis for further changes in the nursing care plan.

When writing an evaluation of the patient, you will need to consider the patient's condition on arrival or when diagnosis was made, the pathologic or psychosocial problem, the nursing diagnosis, expected outcomes, and interventions.

Some questions to ask yourself include the following:

- What are the signs and symptoms of the pathologic problem, psychosocial problem, and nursing diagnosis?
- Which symptoms are present and which are not?
- Are the patient's symptoms stable, worse, or improved?
- How close is the patient to meeting the expected outcome?
- Which interventions are working? Which are not?
- What changes have you seen? What has not changed?

You can collect data for your evaluation statement from:

- Laboratory and x-ray study reports
- Procedure results
- Graphic and flow sheets, including I & Os
- Post-procedure vital sign flow sheets
- Previous professional notes
- Doctor's orders, when parameters are given
- Physical reassessment
- Observations by yourself, other staff members, and family members
- Other available data.

When writing an evaluation progress note, the amount of time reviewed varies depending on the situation and the type of evaluation you are doing. You should be guided by patient acuity, whether the problem is an actual or high risk for problem, hospital or unit standards, or the situation.

In most cases, your work is not finished when you write an evaluation. Based on the results of your evaluation, the patient's care plan may be revised and require one of the following:

- Further assessment of the patient to find the correct diagnosis
- Continuation of the plan of care as written
- Continuation of the plan of care with increased effort
- Modification of the plan of care
- A combination of the above
- Resolution or inactivating of the diagnosis.

Objective and Subjective Information

Evaluative statements are made with objective data. As you read nursing notes, you frequently will see progress notes that make a subjective evaluation. A subjective evaluation does not communicate clearly to the reader. For example, what is the writer saying with these statements?

- Condition worse
- Complaining of pain
- Better day

These comments are frequently used by themselves without any supporting data. They leave the reader to ask:

- How was the patient worse?
- Where was the pain and how severe was it?
- How did the patient have a better day?

You might mean that a patient was "worse" in terms of his activity level, but at the same time he could be in excellent condition regarding pain control or mental status. What did you base your opinion on? There is nothing wrong with the statement "condition worse" if you support that statement with the facts. The following examples compare subjective and objective statements.

*5-7: Evaluative Statement–
Subjective Statements Compared
to Objective Statements*

Subjective Statements	Objective Statements	
Condition worse	Activity Intolerance	DATA: Activity level decreasing each day. Monday was walking in the halls Tuesday tired going to the bathroom. Today states doesn't have the strength to get out of bed.———— RESPONSE: Activity tolerance level decreasing. ———————— *F. Honn RN*
Complaining of pain	Pain	DATA: C/O sudden, severe, sharp, and constant pain in L leg going from groin to toes. States "It hurts for the sheets to touch my leg." Pain rated 10 on scale 1 to10, 10 severe. *R. Wright LPN*
Better day	Pain	DATA: Able to sit up for all three meals for first time since surgery. No nausea and vomiting, yesterday vomited 6 times. Now on po pain medication and has stated that pain is well controlled, medicated for pain twice in last 18 hours. "I feel good today."———————— RESPONSE: Patient stronger and had a better day today than yesterday. *B. Harve LPN*

An objective statement allows the reader to understand exactly what is going on with the patient. Remember, readers have different perspectives. Your job is to make the meaning clear to your reader. Do Exercise 5-2 to practice writing objective statements.

Other subjective statements include comments or words such as the following:

drinking well	lung sounds normal	often
voiding well	patient is anxious	rarely
voiding qs	better	seldom

| good | no difficulty | occasionally |
| frequently | most of the time | a lot |

Evaluate the terms you use to describe a patient. If two people read your note, would they get the same information? Could they make a critical judgment?

Exercise 5-2

Make the following subjective statements objective statements. Create appropriate data to make your statement objective.

Subjective Statement   Objective Statement

Weak

_____

_____

_____

_____

Condition Better

_____

_____

_____

_____

Evaluative statements express your professional opinion, which has been made based on objective data. An evaluative statement can be written in two ways. The evaluative statement can follow the notation of the objective data that supports your opinion. Or, the evaluative statement can immediately precede the support data.

Example 5-8: Evaluative Statement–Judgment Followed by Data

Focus	Progress Note
Nausea	RESPONSE: Tolerating oral fluids well, drank 450cc in last hour and half with not nausea or vomiting. *K. Baird Rn*

Example 5-9: Evaluative Statement–Data Followed by Judgment

Focus	Progress Note
Nausea	RESPONSE: Drank 450cc in last hour and half with no nausea or vomiting. Tolerating oral fluids. *K. Baird Rn*

How you write an evaluative statement often depends on the documentation format you are using. With Focus Charting, the evaluative statement will be made in the RESPONSE component of the note. The narrative format does not provide guidance; either method can be used.

The proper approach to writing an evaluation is to state exactly what is happening, including volumes, amounts, and totals. State exactly what you see, what you did, and how it was done. State the patient's verbal and clinical response to the care rendered.

Examples 5-7 through 5-11 are examples of evaluative statements made in general nursing notes. Some facilities require an evaluative statement on each nursing diagnosis once every 24 hours. These notes can encompass more data. Let's look at several examples.

Example 5-10: Evaluative Statement–of Specific Nursing Diagnosis

Focus	Progress Note
Mobility Impaired	Data: Today able to get out of bed with help of one who needs to support and move R leg. Walked in hall, using walker and escorted by PT tech, for first time post-op. Went 30 feet without becoming diaphoretic, weak, or shaky. "That felt great! It only hurt when I first stood up, but that went away quickly." Had been medicated for pain an hour before ambulating. Sat up in chair for one hour x2. ACTION: Reminded not to bend forward in chair so that hip was at an angle >90 degrees, otherwise has been observing total hip precautions. Continue with care plan with increased activity. RESPONSE: Mobility continues to improve. *F. Honn RN*

The next example involves a change in the care plan because a new problem has been identified that is affecting the original problems. The patient with diabetes has a nonhealing leg ulcer. She smokes, sits in a wheelchair for long periods of time, and eats junk food.

Example 5-11: Evaluative Statement–With Care Plan Revision

Focus	Progress Note
Anxiety	DATA: Has been smoking frequently during the day, admits to 3/4 pack in 6 hours. Has spent 3 1/2 hours on outside porch in wheel chair smoking, with leg in dependent position. When asked about Hostess Twinkies in bedside stand states she has eaten three packages today, and admits eating them frequently when out on porch since admission and at home. "I just take more insulin." Fingerstick blood sugars ranging from 240–354 since admission. Does not look at me when discussing situation, constantly picking at robe, and looking out window. When asked if she was worried became teary eyed, but said no. Was able to get her to talk about her family and life. ————— ACTION: Explained we wanted to help her and that in order for healing to occur she needed to stop smoking, control sugar level, ————————————— (Continued) *R. Wright LPN*

(Continued) | and elevate her leg. Explained availability of counselors to assist. Consult set to Mrs. James, Psychiatry Nurse Practitioner. See care plan.————————————————————————————
RESPONSE: Agreed to talk with Mrs. James and to try not to smoke.———————————————— *R. Wright LPN*

This note clearly demonstrates the way in which nursing documentation can affect patient care. It provides a partial explanation for the elevated blood sugar and the nonhealing ulcer. The identification of this problem can initiate proper interventions by nurses, dietitians, doctors, and diabetic educators and can save this woman suffering, expense, time in the hospital, and probably her foot.

Summary

This chapter has emphasized the following key points:

1. There are four basic types of summaries statements pertaining to patient care: admission, transfer, discharge, and death summaries.
2. In the admission assessment summary, you organize the data obtained from the nursing admission assessment, physical examination, and clinical data and any other patient data.
3. Transfer notes provide continuity of care between the sending and receiving units or facilities. You must communicate why the patient was in your care, what had been done, results of that care, and the reason for transfer.
4. Discharge summaries describe the care given during the patient's hospitalization and identify the patient's status on discharge.
5. Period summaries describe care during a specified time frame. (This manual did not include examples of period summaries.)

6. Evaluative statements are comprised of two parts: objective data, which is measurable and verifiable, and professional judgment.

7. Objective statements allow the reader to understand exactly on what your judgment is based.

8. Do not use subjective, nondescript terms.

Notes:

Chapter 6

Writing Nursing Progress Notes

Objectives

The learner will be able to:
1. Write complete, concise, and clear nursing notes regarding:
   A. Condition changes
   B. Situations or events
   C. Nursing interventions
2. Write notes that reflect the patient's response to interventions.

If any of the information in these notes already appears on flow sheets in your clinical area, you will not need to repeat it in your narrative note. The information is presented here to illustrate data that must be documented on one of these two types of forms.

Documentation of patient care and patient status was summarized in Chapter 5. Also discussed was writing evaluative statements used to document professional evaluation of the patient. This chapter demonstrates how to write nursing progress notes. The discussion is organized into three categories of nursing notes: patient's condition, situation or events, and nursing interventions. When you write daily progress notes, these three categories usually blend together and often are in one nursing note. You need not be concerned about the specific category of information; your job is to get the information on paper.

As a nurse, you will wear many hats and do many different types of jobs. As you document, you are a historian and a journalist. Like a historian, you are reporting retrospective data because you never document before the act or event. When a reporter writes an article, the article must answer the questions who, what, when, where, why, and how. As a nurse you essentially do the same thing, but from the nursing process model, and you often are an active participant in the event. In addition, the note should reflect an accurate chronology of events.

Let's look at an example.

Example 6-1: Reaction to Treatment

Focus	Progress Note
IV site irritation	DATA: C/O pain in R hand @ IV site. Hand reddened from IV site to 1 1/2 inches above site, tender and warm to touch. Afebrile No swelling. —————————————————————— ACTION: IV discontinued and restarted in L forearm, @ 1815, with #18 gauge over-the-needle catheter with one puncture using aseptic technique. Warm moist towel applied to R hand for 15 minutes. Will do warm soaks q4h and monitor site q4h.—————— RESPONSE: "This towel makes my hand feel better." *G. Bass RN*

Now let's analyze this note in relationship to the nursing process.

Assessment: DATA section of the note.
Nursing Diagnosis: IV site irritation. (Remember, all facilities do not use NANDA nursing diagnoses.)
Planning: Immediate plan was to change IV site. Warm soaks and monitoring site.
Interventions: Change IV site and warm moist soaks to old site. Monitoring of old site.
Evaluation: An immediate subjective response is pertinent, but not a major factor in the outcome of the problem. The important

evaluation of the problem takes place in the future, after the full treatment has been in effect.

In most cases, nursing progress notes make up the majority of your nursing documentation. As with any repetitive activity, it is easy to become complacent or overwhelmed with this responsibility. When you are responsible for the care of between 2 and 20 patients, so many events occur that it is difficult to find time to document or to remember what you need to document. Methods that can help you document even when you have a heavy patient load include the following:

- Document as soon as possible after the event.
- Keep notes on your report sheet.
- Use flow sheets to the maximum, when available.
- Do not repeat information documented on flow sheets, unless required to enhance evaluation notes.
- Review Nursing Care Plan.
- Review doctor's orders.
- Review Kardex.
- Review previous nursing notes.

Develop your own memory techniques for documentation that allow you to enhance quality care through appropriate documentation. Whatever system you develop, it must be flexible enough to adapt to different situations but stable enough to be useful.

Patient's Condition

One of your major responsibilities as a nurse, is to identify the patient's ever-changing condition through the use of the nursing process. You finalize the nursing process by documenting your findings so that other team members can have access to the information.

While you document on a patient's record, you have a good opportunity to further evaluate your patient's condition. You have access to notes written by other team members and other clinical data. Many times this additional information clarifies your own findings. Your nursing progress notes can help establish the medical diagnosis or uncover another problem. You may find that further assessment is necessary once you combine the information from other sources with your nursing information.

You will write several types of patient condition notes that show deterioration, improvement, no change, problem resolved, or adverse reactions. Let's look at an example of each type of note.

Condition Deterioration

The Example 6-2 describes a condition deterioration in an elderly surgical patient who starts to develop congestive heart failure.

Example 6-2: Condition Deterioration–Leading to New Nursing Diagnosis

Date/Time Focus	Progress Note
8/23/93 Fluid Volume 0800 Excess	DATA: AM assessment shows the following changes from 2300 assessment. Crackles heard bilaterally with inspiratory wheeze L lower lobe. Now complains of being tired this AM and noticed was slightly dyspneic when going to BR. BP up from 136/86 @ 2200 to 148/96 now, T 99.2°F P 96 R 24. Awoke with moist sounding nonproductive cough. Other assessment parameters unchanged from 2300; see Physical Assessment Flow Sheet. Has history of CHF. ———————— ACTION: Instructed to stay in bed, head of bed elevated 45 degrees. Notified Dr. Wilson of the above changes in lungs sounds, vitals signs, cough, dyspnea, and tiredness. See doctor orders. O_2 @ 2 L/min by nasal cannula started at 0745. EKG, ABGs and blood work done stat, see appropriate reports. Given 40mg IV Lasix and AM digoxin early, see MAR. Instructed on purpose and effects of Lasix. Instructed to call for help to go to BR. Side rails up and call light in reach. Restarted I & O. Do q4h lung assessments. ———————— RESPONSE: Verbalized her intent to call for help as needed. ———————————————— *B. Harve LPN*

Improvement

Because you were observant and reacted quickly, you could document an improvement in her condition after your 1300 reassessment.

Example 6-3: Condition Improvement–After Treatment for Problem Noted in Example 6-2

Date/Time Focus	Progress Note
8/23/93 Fluid Volume 1300 Excess	RESPONSE: No crackles or wheezing heard in lungs on auscultation. BP 136/88 T 98.2°F P 82 R 18. Denies cough, dyspnea, weakness, or tiredness when in bed or up. Output 1500cc since Lasix given. "I feel so much better then I did this morning." Respiratory and circulatory condition improved. ———————————— *B. Harve LPN*

(Remember, a focus narrative note can have one, two, or all three segments of a DAR note.) You gave significant treatment for a serious medical problem. You would normally be watching this patient closely throughout your shift. Watching is not the end of your responsibility; you must document the response achieved. This situation could just as easily result in a further deterioration of the condition.

Sometimes a change in the patient's condition leads to a new nursing diagnosis. Example 6-1 is an excellent illustration. Documentation of a patient's change of condition usually involves the writing of evaluative statements. Such statments should use the guidelines given in Chapter 5. Your daily documentation responsibilities will include documentation of condition changes or writing status reports on active problems. Depending on the seroiusness of the problem, you may need to write more than one note on your shift. Example 6-4 documents a change in condition nursing note, when a patient experiences fewer stools after had multiple diarrhea stools.

Example 6-4: Condition Improvement–Active Problem

Focus	Progress Note
Diarrhea	DATA: Has had 8 liquid brown stools with mucus between 06 and 1500 today. Has only had 2 liquid brown stools with mucus since 1500. States cramping has also decreased and mouth not as dry.————————————————*D. Wilson RN*

No Change

Even though Example 6-3 indicates the patient has apparently returned to her normal condition, this problem must be tracked to ensure it has been properly treated and has resolved. During the next shift, if everything remains stable the following no change in condition note may be written.

Example 6-5: No Change in Condition

Focus	Progress Note
Fluid Volume Excess	DATA: Lungs clear bilaterally on auscultation. No edema of feet, hands, sacrum, or eyelids. Denies dyspnea at rest or when active. No cough. Ambulating twice during shift, 40-60 feet each time, no assistance required. "Except for the fact I had surgery I feel great." ————————————— ACTION: Continue plan of care.————————— RESPONSE: Stable with no signs of active CHF. *F. Honn RN*

Depending on what information is already documented on the physical assessment flow sheet, some of the preceding information need not be restated.

Problem Resolved

Example 6-5 is an evaluative statement and clearly defines the patient's status. The problem could probably be resolved at this time, but it is better to continue to track it for a while. Before resolving this problem, consider the patient's overall health status and risk for further problems with this diagnosis. When you do resolve the problem, your note could be similar to the following:

Example 6-6: Problem Resolved

Focus	Progress Note
Fluid Volume Excess	DATA: For the last 48 hours: Lungs clear bilaterally on auscultation. No edema of feet, hands, sacrum, or eyelids. Denies dyspnea at rest or when active. No cough. Ambulating in halls 4 or 5 times during the day, 40–60 feet each time, no assistance required. Vital signs stable. —————————————————
ACTION: Advised patient to report any recurrence of tiredness, edema, dyspnea, cough, weakness, or any change in condition. Continue shift physical assessment per protocol. Problem resolved.————————————————— *P. Pizzuto LPN*

Adverse Reactions

A patient involved with medical tests or treatments is at risk for developing complications. An adverse reaction to a test or medical treatment must be treated, monitored, and then documented, usually as a new nursing diagnosis. The following note describes a patient who developed a local cellulitis at the site of the injection of IVP dye.

Example 6-7: Adverse Reactions

Focus	Progress Notes
Swollen R Arm	DATA: Awaken @ 0315, complaining of pain in R arm. R arm swollen from 6 inches above and 4 inches below elbow. R elbow 1″ in diameter >L elbow. Has red streak going up arm 6″ starting at puncture site in R antecubital area. T 99.8°F. No drainage from puncture site. Arm tender to touch. Reports that puncture site is where IVP dye was injected yesterday AM. Pain 8 on scale 1–10, 10 worse.—————————————————
ACTION: Arm elevated on pillows. Notified Dr. Whitacre of the above assessment, see doctor's orders. Moist heat applied with K-pad. IV ampicillin started and Darvon given, see MAR. Placed on q4h vitals, pain medicate prn, assess swelling q4h, and moist soaks and antibiotics as ordered. Explained purpose of moist heat, elevation and antibiotics. Instructed patient to report any further problems and request pain medication as needed.
RESPONSE: Pain now 4, on scale of 1-10. *S. Estever RN*

105

Situations or Events
Refusal of Treatment

The days of automatic patient compliance with physicians' recommendations are over. Patients are now consumers of health care. They demand to know what the health team is doing and why. Law and health care ethics give the competent patient the right to make informed decisions and to refuse care. They may refuse treatments even if it endangers their life.

In some cases the patient or family refused a prescribed treatment because of inadequate information about the purpose of the test or treatment. The nurse must always ensure that the patient who refuses a treatment or test has appropriate information.

What would you do if the patient refused to take a bowel prep before a barium enema? Your first step is to find out why the patient refused and then to provide education about the need for the prep and the rationale for the barium enema. If the patient still refused treatment, a note documenting the refusal might look like the following:

Example 6-8: Refusal of Treatment

Focus	Progress Note
Refusal of Barium Enema Prep	DATA: Refused to take bowel prep for barium enema. "I don't need any more tests. I don't know why the doctor ordered it."_____ ACTION: Expiained the importance of test to diagnoses current problems, difficulty of treating him properly if diagnosis not made definitively, and importance of having bowels properly cleared. Allowed patient to ventilate anger, frustrations, and fears. Dr. Giraroud notified of patient's refusal; he will talk with patient on evening rounds. Prep held._____ RESPONSE: Refused barium enema prep. *K. Baird RN*

As stated earlier, a patient has a right to refuse any test or treatment. You must show that you provided information regarding the need for the intervention. If the patient continues to refuse the test or treatment you also must indicate that you did not perform the intervention.

Patient Injury

A patient injury is a serious situation. It may be related to an action by the patient, by equipment failure, or by staff actions. You need to indicate clearly what happened without blaming or finger pointing. You need to report the facts of what happened, what was done to correct the problem, and the results of the injury and treatment. One of the most frequent causes of injury is a patient fall.

Example 6-9: Patient Injury

Focus	Progress Note
Patient found on floor	DATA: Patient heard calling out and was found on carpeted floor beside bed @ 0213. "I had a hard time getting down that pipeline." Was at foot of bed, all four bed rails up, call light within reach, soft safety vest was still secured to bed without patient in it. Rubbing R hip. Obvious deformity noted on R hip, R foot rotated out, and R leg shorter then L. Bilateral pedal pulses strong, capillary refill in feet <3 sec, feet warm and pink, able to move toes. Unable to assess numbness, tingling, pain, or exactly what happened since patient remains disoriented to person, place, and time. BP 148/96 P 112 R 18. Skin intact.————— ACTION: Placed on backboard and then on stretcher. Notified Mrs. Morton, Nursing Supervisor, and Dr. Wilford of the above incident and assessment, see doctor's orders. To x-ray at 0225 and returned @ 0245, x-ray shown R hip fracture. Meperidine and promethazine HCL IM given @ 0250, see MAR. Dr. Wilford notified Mrs. Dowton, patient's guardian, of fracture, Mrs. Dowton arrived to sign consent for surgery at 0330. IV started with #18 gauge angio catheter in L forearm, D_5W infusing at 100cc per hour. See pre-op flow sheet and MAR for pre-op prep. To OR at 0335 via stretcher.————— RESPONSE: Vitals, taken q15min after fall, remain stable; see flow sheet. *K. Baird RN*

After you take care of the immediate patient needs, an occurrence screen or incident or variance report must be completed. I cannot stress too strongly that you DO NOT document the fact that you wrote a report in the patient's chart. An occurrence screen or incident or variance report is the property of the hospital and is used to investigate the situation and to report to risk management. By documenting the existence of the report in the patient's chart, you have made the report discoverable (giving the patient's lawyer access to the report in the event of legal action).

Telephone Calls

Besides calls to doctors, other calls are sometimes necessary to facilitate patient care. For example, I had to call the nursing home from which a patient had just been transferred to find out about previous immunizations. The note read something like this:

Example 6-10: Telephone Call

Focus	Progress Note
Immunization Assessment	ACTION: Called Mrs. Clark, RN Nursing Supervisor of Bay Manor Nursing Home to verify if patient has previously received Pneumovac immunization. She reports his immunization records show he had the vaccination on 8/25/92. Vaccination not given, MAR so annotated. *S. Estever RN*

In another example the anesthesiologist had to be notified on a weekend that a patient had been admitted for surgery on Monday.

Example 6-11: Telephone Call

Focus	Progress Note
(Excerpt from admission assessment)	ACTION: Notified Dr. Murphy, duty anesthesiologist, patient was on ward, had sinuses congestion, moist nonproductive cough, and a cousin with history of malignant hyperthermia. *F. Honn RN*

Occurrence of Error

Sometimes nurses give the wrong medication or make other types of mistakes that must be reported. For example, if you gave Demerol and Phenergan and the order read Demerol and Vistaril, the note would read as follows:

Example 6-12: Occurrence of Error

Focus	Progress Note
Medication administration	DATA: C/O pain in R knee, rated as 10. Pain constant and sharp Could not get comfortable. 1345 vitals: BP 124/82 P 92 R 16. NKDA. Alert & oriented to person, place, and time. Pain rated as 6 @ 1345. ———————————————————————— ACTION: Given Demerol and Phenergan @ 1315, see MAR, for pain. Notified Mrs. Lee, RN, Head Nurse and Dr. James. No orders.———————————————————————— RESPONSE: Obtaining relief from pain. *D. Wilson RN*

You would then document the Demerol and Phenergan injection as a single dose medication on the MAR. Once again you would write up an occurrence screen, incident, or variance report, without noting that fact on the patient's record. Most notes about pain would not indicate vital signs or allergy history. They are included in Example 6-12 as part of the patient assessment after administration of a nonordered medication.

In this note, the pain was rated on a scale of 1 to 10, 10 being most severe. If there is no standard for rating pain, you will need to document what scale you are using, because some people use a 1 to 5 and others use a 1 to 10 scale.

Interventions

What are nursing interventions? *Mosby's Medical, Nursing, and Allied Health Dictionary* defines a nursing intervention as:

> ...Any act by a nurse that implements the nursing care plan or any specific objective of that plan, such as turning a comatose patient to

avoid the development of decubitus ulcers or teaching injection technique to a patient with diabetes before discharge from the hospital. The patient may require intervention in the form of support, limitation, medication, or treatment for the current condition or to prevent the development of further stress. As stress increases, the need to adapt and the need for nursing intervention increases.[1]

Occasionally, you must document what others have done because they may not have documentation responsibilities. In that case make sure you indicate who did the event or whose observations you are reporting.

Example 6-13: Recording Observations of Other Staff Members

Focus	Progress Note
Ambulation	DATA: Dangled on side of bed for ten minutes at 2015, supervised by M. Kelley, NA, who reports patient had no weakness, dyspnea, diaphoresis, or nausea. *P. Pizzuto LPN*

Example 6-14: Recording Patient's Observations

Focus	Progress Note
Ambulation	DATA: Dangled on side of bed for ten minutes at 2015, supervised by M. Kelley, NA. Patient later reported to me she had no weakness, dyspnea, diaphoresis, or nausea. *P. Pizzuto LPN*

As you can see from the preceding definition, almost anything can be considered an act of implementation. Your responsibility is to document those acts or events that have a significant impact on the patient's well-being. The trick is to know what should and should not be documented. Events that should be documented were identified in Chapter 4.

Implementation of the care plan will be documented in several different ways. Some items, such as routine care and use of equipment, are often documented on flow sheets. Monitoring activities, such as frequent vital signs, circulatory checks, IV fluid administration, intracranial pressure readings, and Swan-Ganz catheter readings are tracked on flow sheets or graphs.

Occasionally, you will summarize information on the flow sheet in a narrative note. Each hospital has its own flow sheets to facilitate documentation of routine care, monitoring activities, or other activities such as wound care and shift physical assessment. You will use these flow or graphic sheets for the basic documentation, but they will never cover all of your documentation responsibilities. For example, if when doing the physical assessment you note that personnel on the last three shifts reported that the lungs were clear on auscultation, but you now hear crackles, a narrative note is indicated. Your narrative note should indicate your new findings, the assessment of the change, what you did to resolve the situation, patient teaching, your plan of care, and the results of your action. Flow sheets facilitate documentation, but the use of flow sheets does not alleviate documentation responsibilities. Nor does it prevent you from using data from a flow sheet when writing an evaluative or implementation statement.

> To repeat some of the information in these notes may already appear on flow sheets in your clinical area. In this case you will not need to repeat it in your narrative note. The information is here to illustrate required data that must be documented either on flow sheets or in a narrative note.

Unscheduled Medications

One area often ignored when documenting is the response to one-time medications. In Example 6-2, Lasix was given as a one-time order to correct a problem due to congestive heart failure. Response was clearly documented in the note for the 1300 assessment. You must remember the reason for administering a medication and its expected effects. What were the results? Did it resolve the problem? You must document the patient's response to the medication.

Another example of an unscheduled medication would be giving a laxative for constipation postoperatively. The patient had no bowel prep before surgery and has been confined to bed rest after surgery.

Example 6-15: Unscheduled Medications

Focus	Progress Note
Constipation	DATA: Has had no BM for 3 days, on bed rest, and is on regular diet. C/O slight nausea and abdominal discomfort. Bowel sounds present.——————————————————— ACTION: Given MOM. Instructed to drink at least 8 glasses of H$_2$O each day and select food with fiber. Encouraged to continue turning q2h. *G. Bass RN*

Because a patient would not have a response to the Milk of Magnesia (MOM) for several hours, it will probably be the responsibility of the next shift to document the response. The response should read something like the following.

Example 6-16: Response to Unscheduled Medications

Focus	Progress Note
Constipation	RESPONSE: Had large, brown, formed BM. "I feel so much better Thanks!" *R. Wright LPN*

Spiritual Interventions

Religious events or ceremonies should be documented because many patients and their family find strength and comfort from them, which enhances their recovery and well-being. Sometimes religious ceremonies are performed when the patient is unaware of the event, such as Sacrament of the Sick. A patient's spiritual well-being can be an essential component in a seemingly impossible recovery. Nurses have learned never to underestimate the power of a person's spiritual beliefs.

An example of documentation regarding spiritual intervention follows:

Example 6-17: Spiritual Interventions

Focus	Progress Note
Sacrament of the sick	DATA: Patient has been unconscious since admission, after being found on the side of the road. Has not been identified. Only possession found on patient was a broken rosary. Condition guarded.——————————————————— ACTION: At 1515 notified Father Donovan of St. Lukes Catholic Church of above information and requested that he administer Sacrament of the Sick if it is appropriate. Father Donovan agreed that ceremony was appropriate and would be on ward within the hour. ——————————————— *D. Wilson RN*

Because the above notation was made right after the call, a second note is required.

Example 6-18: Spiritual Interventions

Focus	Progress Note
Sacrament of the sick	ACTION: Father Donovan administered Sacrament of the Sick. Will make daily visits and advised us to call when the patient's condition changes. Care plan has been updated. Patient remains unconscious.——————————————— *D. Wilson RN*

Patient Teaching

Being in the hospital is a very scary experience, partially because the patient is faced with many unknowns: Will I recover? Will there be changes in my life-style? Will there be pain? Will I be able to pay for this hospitalization? Fear of the unknown can be incapacitating or at the very least disruptive to a person's life-style. Think about the last time you were faced with an unknown. Did you sleep well? How often did thoughts of that unknown disrupt your rest?

One way to decrease fear of the unknown is to educate your patient. Patient education is also used to help the patient make informed decisions and to ensure the ability to do self-care.

Let's look at a note for patient teaching regarding self-catheterization.

Example 6-19: Patient Teaching

Focus	Progress Note
Patient Teaching Self-Cath	DATA: Voided 250cc at 0850 and catheterized at 0855 for a post residual of 350cc of clear yellow urine.———————— ACTION: Initiated self-catheterization teaching. Goal was for patient to explain why self-catheterization is necessary, and observe a catheterization. Explained reason for self-catheterization post MMK. Given handout "Self-Catheterization" (NF 245/93) to read. Explained difference between clean technique and sterile technique for catheterization. Explained importance of doing catheterization within 30 minutes of voiding. I performed sterile catheterization with mirror propped so patient could observe. After next void patient to demonstrate self-catheterization and catheter care.———————— RESPONSE: Stated why self-catheterization necessary. Asked relevant questions during procedure and was able to identify meatus with use of mirror. Now reading handout. *F. Honn RN*

Remember, patients are not always ready to hear what you have to tell them. Some of the things you have to teach the patient may be repugnant to them. For example, after you have been a nurse for several years giving an injection is not difficult, but to patients, giving themselves injections can be a major problem. What did you do to move the patient toward the necessary education or alleviate the patient's fears? Document that the patient is not ready to learn, why (if known), and your interventions. You may need to open a new nursing diagnosis to address the problem.

In some cases, you may need to teach the patient's spouse, guardian, or significant other how to perform the self-care. If a wife does all the cooking, she will need to be involved with dietary instructions with the husband. Think about who will have to perform the task. Will they need help? Who is the patient's support system?

Lack of Understanding

Example 6-20: Lack of Patient Understanding

The last example describes a situation in which a patient and his family put the patient at risk of injury.

Focus	Progress Note
Patient Education: Traction	DATA: Found patient in bed with skeletal traction removed. When questioned states family removed the traction because it bothered him, it was painful, and he did not want to be "hung up anymore". C/O pain rated as a 6, scale of 1–10 (10 worse), Circulatory check remains unchanged from assessment documented 1/2 hour ago. ACTION: Notified Dr. Good of traction removal by family, he will be in to talk with patient and reapply traction. With the help of Mrs. Sanchez, Spanish interpreter, explained reasons for traction to patient and family including stabilization of bones, prevention of complications, help the healing process, and decrease pain until surgery tomorrow. Explained if he was in pain we could give him medicine for the pain and that doctor will be in to talk with him. Made flash cards in English and Spanish for pain, shot, pills, and other words to facilitate communication. Medicated with IM Demerol & Phenergan at 2130, see MAR.——————————— RESPONSE: Mrs. Sanchez states family stated that they thought pain was from the weights and they promise to talk with staff when they do not understand or have a question. *B. Harve LPN*

This note illustrates several types of interventions: communication with patient and family, pain control, prn medication, and education. In addition to recording those interventions, you also document telephone communications and any situation in which patient and family action could potentially contribute to a patient injury. When the patient and family have limited understanding of English, the use of an interpreter is important to enhance understanding, decrease suspicions, and gain cooperation. The documentation of the use of the interpreter is important to demonstrate your continuing commitment to providing quality care and meeting your responsibilities.

115

Summary

This chapter has emphasized the following key points:

1. Daily progress notes must answer the questions who, what, when, where, why, and how.
2. Each note should indicate all or most elements of the nursing process.
3. Progress notes must address improvement, deterioration, or no change in condition.
4. A nursing note should be a clear picture of the patient's condition or the event being documented.

Reference

1. Glanze, W.D. (Ed.). (1990). *Mosby's Medical, Nursing, and Allied Health Dictionary*. St. Louis: Mosby-Year Book, 826.

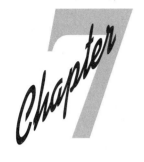

Chapter 7

Using Flow Sheets and Other Forms

Objectives

The learner will be able to:
1. Explain the use of flow sheets and other forms.
2. List five uses of flow sheets and other forms.

It is impossible to illustrate exactly what forms you will see in the clinical setting, examples in this chapter are parts of various forms you will deal with.

Although the goal of this manual is to teach you how to write clear, complete, and concise nursing notes, documentation on flow sheets and other types of forms is also part of your responsibilities. This chapter describes several types of forms that you may work with in clinical practice. Flow sheets and other forms used to document patient care are not standardized but rather vary from agency to agency and often within an agency. The main similarity is the use of several different styles of form design. The forms used in this chapter have been designed specifically for this manual and are based on many different examples. Because it is impossible to illustrate exactly what you will see in the clinical setting, examples in this chapter are parts of various forms you will deal with.

Over the years nurses have endeavored to meet their documentation requirements in an environment of increasingly sicker patients, decreasing staff, and advancing technology.

After considering the documentation requirements, nurses developed flow sheets to handle the documentation of repetitive and day-to-day tasks that need no explanation and to decrease the number of different forms. The latter is accomplished by placing many different forms on larger sheets of paper that are then folded and placed in the record. Other forms have been designed to cover important events to ensure that the event is appropriately documented. All of the forms of a particular documentation system are important to the documentation of a patient's health status while under your care. Each form must be completed accurately and in detail.

Flow sheets are used to document I & O, activity of daily living, safety, wound monitoring, data of monitoring activities, and physical assessments. Other types of forms include patient education, admission assessments, and discharge summaries. While using any flow sheet or other form remember that they:

- Do not release you from appropriate narrative documentation of events such as those noted in Chapters 4, 5, and 6.
- Cannot always address everything about a subject.
- Are not always appropriate for a particular situation.
- Sometimes need to be supported by narrative notes.
- Must be used correctly, as directed by policies and procedures.

Remember, too, that these forms are used to support but not totally replace narrative documentation.

The basic guidelines and rules used for narrative documentation are also true for documenting on flow sheets and other forms. One major problem with these forms is that staff will often use unapproved abbreviations to try to say everything in a very small space. If you have more to say then fits in the space, document the information in the progress notes; do not use unapproved abbreviations.

Common Features

Even though forms are not standardized everywhere, they have several common features:

- Date and time when the form was used to record patient information
- Area to verify initials
- Hospital identification and form name or number (The form name usually identifies form's use.)
- Patient identification

A typical form (Example 7-1) will have a way to identify the chart form and patient at either the top or bottom of each form. Make sure to stamp each form with the patient's imprint plate; check to see that it can be read clearly. Check this area before documenting on the record to ensure that you have the proper form and proper record.

Example 7-1: Chart Form and Patient Identification

Patient Identification	**Patient Memorial Hospital** Tipp City, Ohio **Activities of Daily Living Flow Sheet**

Somewhere on each form will be an area similar to Example 7-2, Initial Verification. This section allows each set of initials to be matched to the specific person who documented information. Make sure that someone else can read your signature. Credentials identify whether you are a student, an RN, or an LPN.

Example 7-2: Initial Verification

Signatures of Staff	
Initials	Signatures/Credentials

Admission Assessment

The form for the admission assessment varies depending on the patient population. You will usually find a different assessment form for adults, pediatric, psychiatry, intensive care, and labor and delivery. How the assessment is completed also varies. Some institutions allow the patient to document part of the information and the staff to review and complete the form. Others require the staff to complete the entire form. In either case you must be sure that the form is as accurate as possible. The term *as possible* is used here because patients have been known to tell the nurse one thing and the doctor something else.

During the completion of an admission assessment, you are collecting a database so that you can:

- Make the appropriate nursing diagnosis.
- Identify possible causes or contributing factors to the problem(s).
- Identify areas of preventive health care that the patient needs to address, such as self-breast or self-testicular examinations, PAP tests, well-baby care, and immunizations.
- Identify teaching needs.
- Identify potential problems on discharge.
- Start discharge planning.
- Have a better understanding of your patient.

An effective admission assessment is long and will take time to complete, so plan accordingly. Example 7-3, Admission Assessment[1] is part of a complete assessment that includes types of questions that could be asked during an admission assessment.

After looking at Example 7-3, which is an incomplete assessment, it will be evident that a large volume of data is obtained about the patient. This information is used to write the admission summary. All of the information obtained is not used in the admission summary, but it is available for later review. A day rarely goes by that I do not refer back to the admission assessment on a patient.

Example 7-3: Admission Assessment (This example shows only part of the assessment.)

So that we can give you the best care possible while in the hospital and plan for your discharge please complete this form. If you have any questions your nurse will be glad to assist you. These questions are to help us provide you the nursing care you need. Some questions are very personal, but we are required to ask them and we will protect your privacy. Please check the correct answer or provide the information requested.

PART 1.

Date: _____ & Time: _____ of admission. Your age is: ___ Your are: ___ Male ___ Female
Person providing information: ___ Patient
            ___ Other : Name _____ Relationship: _____
            Telephone number: _____

Admitted from: ___ Home   ___ Nursing Home (Name: _____)
          ___ Emergency Room   ___ Doctor's Office (Dr.: _____)
                              ___ Other (Where: _____)

Description of Current Problem
1. What illness or problem caused you to come to the hospital? _____
   _____

2. Describe the events leading to your hospitalization. _____
   _____
   _____
   _____

3. What relieved your symptoms? _____
   _____

What community services do you currently use: ___ Homemaker Aide   ___ Transportation
                                             ___ Physical Therapy   ___ Meals on Wheels
                                             ___ Home Health Agency (Name: _____)
                                             ___ Other (_____)   ___ None

Do you use:
     Alcohol: ___ No, ___ Yes; Type and amount: _____
     Street Drugs: ___ No, ___ Yes; Type and amount: _____

Smoke: ___ No, ___ Yes:

Type: ___ Cigarettes

___ Cigars   ___ Number packs per day

___ Chew   ___ Number of years smoked or chewed

___ Pipe

Main Language: ___ English, ___ Spanish, ___ Other (Which: _____)

Last grade of formal schooling: _____

Preventive Health Care (Dates of Last)

Examination	How Often	Last One
Physical Exam		
Eye Exam		
Dental Exam		
Self-Testicular Exam		
Self-Breast Exam		
Pap Smear		
Mammogram		

Disposition of Medications

___ Not brought to hospital

___ Sent home with (_____)

___ Sent to pharmacy

Perscription medications:

Medication/Dosage	Freqency	Last Dose	Are you Following Dr's Orders	
			Yes	No

Over the counter medications:

Drug	Frequency	Last Dose

Assistive Devices: Location: Hospital   Home

Dentures: ___ No ___ Yes: ___Full ___ Partial (___Upper ___ Lower)   ___   ___

Glasses: ___ No___   ___   ___

Contact Lens: ___ No ___ Yes: ___   ___

Hearing Aid: ___ No ___ Yes: ___ Left, ___ Right, ___ Both Ears   ___   ___

Prosthesis: ___ No ___ Yes: What: _____   ___   ___

Equipment Used:

___ Wheelchair, ___ Cane, ___ Walker, ___ Hospital Bed, ___ Side Rails, ___ Oxygen

___ Bedside Commode, ___ Trapeze Bar, ___ Electrical Recliner Lift Bed, ___ None

What equipment did you bring to the hospital?_____

Part II. Nursing Staff to Complete.

Admitting Diagnosis: _____

T: _____ P: _____ R: _____ B/P R: ____/____ L: ____/____ Ht: _____ inches   Wt: _____ Kg

Language Barrier: ___ No, ___ Yes (Explain _____)

Oriented to: ___ Call Light,   ___ Bathroom,   ___ Side Rails,   ___ Visiting Hours,

___ Visitor Policy,   ___ Telephone,   ___ Mealtimes,   ___ Smoking Policy,

___ Air Conditioning/Heat

Valuables: ___ No ___ Yes; Disposition: ___ Sent Home (Name _____) ____ Safe, #_____,
       ___ Patient Retained (List: _____
_____)

Transportation: ___ Ambulatory, ___ Wheelchair, ___ Stretcher, ___ Other (Specify _____)
Transported by: ___ Transporter, ___ Professional Staff, ___ Other (Specify _____)

Signature of Staff Member completing Part II.
_____ Date: _____ Time: _____

Part III: To be completed by RN only.
RN completed physical assessment prior to finishing Part III? ___ Yes, ___ No (Explain _____
_____)
Patient expresses any concerns regarding hospitalization (fears, financial, self-care, etc.) ___ No ___ Yes (Explain __
_____
_____)

Teaching needs identified and care plan initiated on:
    ___ Orientation to Environment
    ___ Test Procedures (As tests are ordered.)
    ___ Preoperative/Postoperative Teaching
    ___ Diet Management (Diet _____)
    ___ Wound/Ostomy Care
    ___ _____
    ___ _____
    ___ _____

Nursing Diagnosis:
    ___ _____
    ___ _____
    ___ _____

The nurse has reviewed this information and the initial plan of care with me and/or us.
Patient's Signature _____ Date _____ Time _____
Significant Other _____ Date _____ Time _____
RN Signature _____ Date _____ Time _____

Example 7-3 is designed so that the patient or family would complete Part I. Part II can be completed by an LPN or a nursing assistant. Part III must be completed by an RN, as dictated by the Nurse Practice Act of your state, which makes the RN responsible for nursing diagnosis.

Each admission assessment will vary, but your responsibilities are the same:

- Make sure the assessment is accurate and complete.
- Maintain patient privacy.

123

- Provide quality patient care.
- Complete the assessment within the time limits set by the policy and procedures of your facility.
- Initiate any consults on admission that are appropriate. For example, consult the discharge planner for the elderly person who lives alone and was just admitted with a fractured hip after falling.

Flow Sheets

Flow sheets are used to document patient information in many different situations. They were designed to help staff remember what they need to document and to make that documentation easier. Flow sheets routinely provide several choices. You place your initials or a check or write a brief statement in the area provided. Many facilities are now keeping flow sheets and graphs at the bedside or by the room door, allowing the nurse to document as soon as the work is completed. Who (RN, LPN, or nurses assistant) can document on the flow sheet depends on the purpose of the form and the facility policy.

Flow sheets can be a trap for nurses if they are not completed correctly. Avoid the following practices:

- Not paying attention to what you are charting. It is easy to become lax and not chart correct information. This happens when a nurse blindly puts initials in the same area as the nurse on the previous shift. Remember to read what you are signing.
- Underrating the importance of flow sheet documentation to the patient's care and to meeting legal protection needs.
- Depending too much on flow sheets to fulfill all of your documentation responsibilities.

Example 7-4, #1 and #2, Activity of Daily Activities illustrates two different designs of flow sheets: #1 does not provide a space to indicate times that the event was completed;

#2 allows the nurse to document under the hour the event was completed. The extra spaces below "Oral Care q4h" allow the nurse to write in other procedures under the appropriate general heading. Activity of Daily Living flow sheets usually include some or all of the following areas: hygiene, activity, diet, feeding, elimination, safety, risk, IV monitoring, treatments, monitoring, and equipment. Equipment usage is often placed on flow sheets to help ensure reimbursement for its use because, as stated before, correct charging for an item is not sufficient to guarantee reimbursement. You must show usage of the equipment.

Various flow sheet designs offer different advantages. Example 7-4, #1 allows you to see and evaluate how a patient progresses up or down the health continuum over five days. A patient may start out requiring a total bed bath and progress to self-care. Example 7-4, #2, provides better evidence of the timing of events.

Example 7-4: #1 Activity of Daily Living

	Date:															
	Time:	N	D	E	N	D	E	N	D	E	N	D	E	N	D	E*
Hygiene	Self-Bathe															
	Assist Bath															
	Total Bed Bath															
	Shave															
	Shampoo															
	Dental Care															
	Oral Care q4h															

*N=nights D=days E=evenings

Example 7-4: #2 Activity of Daily Living

	Date:																				
	Time:	00	01	02	03	04	05	06	07	08	09		15	16	17	18	19	20	21	22	23
	Self-Bathe																				
	Assist Bath																				

Use of physical assessment flow sheets is becoming more popular in the clinical area. Physical assessment flow sheets take the nurse through a basic review of systems. They allow the busy nurse to document the patient's condition quickly and accurately, usually at the start of the shift, and reduce the amount of narrative documentation required. They also attempt to ensure consistency of documented information about the patient's condition from shift to shift, day to day, and nurse to nurse. Any deviation from normal or major change in a patient's condition must be addressed in the progress notes. Any change in the patient's condition that occurs after the assessment that is documented on the flow sheet must also be documented on the progress notes. (When you need to document further information, most policies and procedures require the nurse to put an asterisk in that field to refer the reader to the progress notes.) Physical assessment flow sheets take on several different forms as shown in Example 7-5, #1 and #2.

Example 7-5: #1 Physical Assessment

		Date:												
		Shift:	N	D	E	N	D	E	N	D	E	N	D	E
		Time:												
Skin	Temperature: 1 Warm, 2 Cool, 3 Cold 4 Hot													
	Moisture: 1 Dry, 2 Damp, 3 Diaphoretic													
	Color: 1 Patient's Norm, 2 Pale, 3 Flushed, 4 Ashen, 5 Cyanotic, 6 Jaundice, 7 _____ , 8 _____													
	Color Status: 1 Unchanged, 2 Improving, 3 Deteriorating													

Example 7-5: #2 Physical Assessment

		Date:			
		Shift:	2300-0700	0700-1500	1500-2300
		Time:			
Skin	Temperature				
	Moisture				
	Color				

Each area on the assessment must be addressed. Example 7-5, #1, a patient's condition can be observed over a period of time, but this form limits your response. Example 7-5, #2, allows the nurse to document what was seen, but this option decreases consistency between notations because nurses respond differently and often use their own personal shorthand notations.

Another type of flow sheet is designed to document repeated or serial assessment data. These include the documentation of frequent vital signs, neurologic assessment, Swan-Ganz catheter reading, serial laboratory results, and fingerstick blood sugar readings. Chapter 3 illustrated the documentation of three sets of vital signs in the various formats of nurses notes. You can see how they tend to clutter the note. You must decide whether it would cause more confusion to document several sets of vital signs in the progress note or use another form to document the vital signs. Example 7-6, Post-procedure Vital Signs, is one design for the frequent documentation of vital signs. This form allows the reviewer to monitor the patient's vital signs and identify any trends so that any problem can be dealt with quickly.

Example 7-6: Post-procedure Vital Signs

Date: ___/___/___ (MM/DD/YR) Procedure: _____					
Time	B/P	Temp	Pulse	Resp	Comments

Example 7-7, Wound Assessment, illustrates one way to monitor wound healing.

Almost any type of situation can be turned into a flow sheet. The development and use of flow sheets depend on many variables such as desire to save time, frequency a task is performed, difficulty tracking the results, and attempting to

127

resolve problems with documentation of a particular type of situation. You may have to use several different forms to document patient information. Make them work for you by looking at them as a means of evaluating your patient. Most forms should be kept at the bedside to provide ease in documentation and evaluation of the patient.

Example 7-7: Wound Assessment

Date: Time:				
Dressing: (Inspected or Changed)				
Dressing Type:				
Type of Skin Closure:				
Condition of Site: (Color, heat, swelling, tenderness, edges approximated)				
Drainage: (Color & Amount)				

Other Forms

Other forms for use in the clinical setting include transfer forms, discharge summaries, discharge instructions, postoperative telephone reports, postoperative assessment, and codes. These forms are designed to ensure that particular information is addressed and communicated. Example 7-8, Postoperative Telephone Report, is used by the ward staff to take a telephone report from the Post Anesthesia Care Area (PACU) staff about a patient returning from surgery.

Conclusion

Flow sheets and other forms can be used in the clinical setting in many different ways. Although forms differ from agency to agency, your responsibility is the same: to document the facts accurately, consistently, and completely in a timely manner to ensure complete documentation of the

*Example 7-8: Post-operative
Telephone Report*

Postoperative Telephone Report

Date/Time Report Called: _____ PACU nurse: _____

Patient: _____

Procedure: _____

Type of anesthesia: _____

Vital signs: B/P: _____ T: _____ P: _____ R: _____

O_2 saturation: _____ on ___ room air or ___ O_2 at ___liters/min via _____

Intake: po: _____   Output: emesis: _____   NG:_____

       IV: _____   urinary: _____   Hemovac: _____

       Other: _____   EBL: _____   JP drain: _____

                                              Other: _____

IV Fluid hanging: _____ carryover: _____cc

Medications with times and dosages:

1. _____

2. _____

3. _____

4. _____

Mental Status: _____

Dressing: _____
_____

Tubes: _____

Equipment: _____

X-ray/Labs completed in PACU: _____

Problems while in PACU: _____
_____

Additional comments:

ETA to ward: _____

Signature of staff member taking report: _____

health status and care of the patient. Follow the policy and procedure for the use of each form and know what it means to check or initial each box. Follow the basic documentation guidelines outlined in Chapter 4.

Summary

This chapter has emphasized the following key points:

1. Flow sheets are used to document repetitive and day-to-day tasks that need no explanation and to decrease the number of different forms.
2. Flow sheets do not release you from the responsibility of writing nursing progress notes.
3. You use the same basic guidelines when documenting on flow sheets and other forms, such as when writing progress notes.
4. Flow sheets are used to document patient data such as vital signs, I & O, activities of daily living, physical assessment, and serial laboratory results.
5. Other forms you may use include nursing admission assessment, discharge assessments, discharge summaries, and postoperative assessments.

Reference

1. Wayne Memorial Hospital. (1991). *Nursing Admission Assessment*. Jesup, GA: Unpublished form.

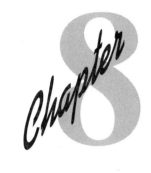

Test

Answer the following questions to the best of your ability. If you cannot answer the question look up the information in the indicated chapter. Then after answering all questions, refer to Chapter 9 for the answers.

Chapter 1

1. According to the ANA's definition of nursing, nurses diagnosis and treat the _____ to actual or potential health problems.

2. You document to meet the needs of whom?

   A._____

   B._____

   C._____

3. The first reason you document is to _____

   _____

4. List six other reasons you document.

A._____

B._____

C._____

D._____

E._____

F._____

5. Why is it important to document the patient's response to the care that has been given? _____

_____

6. True or false. You will be sued because you documented poorly. _____

7. Patients sue nursing professionals because they have

_____

8. True or false. Third-party payers will reimburse the hospital for any supplies as long as they are properly charged for. _____ If false what must you do to ensure proper reimbursement? _____

_____

9. What professional organization sets standards of care for nurses?_____

_____

10. You are given legal permission to work as a nurse by _____, which is administered by the _____, and both are created under _____.

11. What organization surveys a hospital to see whether the institution is meeting established standards? _____

_____

12. If your institution does not pass the above survey what is the impact on the institution? _____

_____

13. What are the standards called that are written by your institution? _____

14. True or False. Abbreviations are universal and any abbreviation may be used in any institution or agency you work in. _____

15. What regulatory agencies mandate your documentation responsibilities? _____

_____

Chapter 2

16. Your practice is defined and based on the _____

_____ process.

17. List the components of the process and what occurs in each step.

A._____

_____

B._____

_____

C._____

_____

D._____

_____

E._____

_____

18. Name the form on which you document patient information on admission to your institution._____

_____

19. On what form do you document all components of the process?_____

20. True or false. Your nursing diagnosis must indicate a need for nursing care. _____ If false, what should it indicate?_____

21. After making a diagnosis, you must _____ it with the patient. Why?_____

_____

22. Identify which component of the process is addressed in the following notes?

Explained the importance of and demonstrated the use of the incentive spirometer._____

Abdomen soft, bowel sounds present, passing flatus.

_____

23. A NANDA Nursing Diagnosis can address which two types of problems?

A. _____

B. _____

24. The following are two NANDA Nursing Diagnoses. If they are correct as written, write "correct" in the space. If they are incorrect, rewrite them.

    A. Noncompliance related to ignorance. _____

    _____

    B. Fear related to unfamiliarity with hospitals.

    _____

25. Indicate which of the following guidelines for writing NANDA nursing diagnosis are incorrect.

    A. Focus on a nurse's task._____

    B. The second part of diagnosis identifies the factors that are believed to be causing or contributing to the problem.

    _____

    C. A single symptom can be used as the human response part of the diagnosis.

    _____

Chapter 3

26. List four different formats of nursing documentation.

    A. _____

    B. _____

    C. _____

    D. _____

27. In which documentation format would you find the following type of notes?

A. D: Wound drainage light green with a foul odor, edge of wound black. Temperature 100.9°F.
A: Sterile dressing done. Old dressing 3/4 saturated with light green drainage.

A. _____

B. S: I have trouble getting my breath.
O: R 26 using accessory muscles with respiration. Crackles heard both lower lobes. T 101.4°F.
A: Ineffective breathing patterns
P: Elevate head of bed, call Dr., push fluids, incentive spirometer q1h.

B. _____

28. Which documentation system sets Standards of Practice and requires the nurse to document only if the patient falls outside of the established norm? _____

_____

29. Explain what each letter of the acronym SOAP means and what type of information is documented in that section of a SOAP note.

S:_____

_____

O:_____

_____

A:_____

_____

P:_____

_____

30. A Focus note is divided into three parts: date/time, the focus, and the progress note. What are the three components of a Focus progress note, and what information is documented in each section?

A._____

_____

B._____

_____

C._____

_____

31. True or false. Every Focus progress note must contain all three components (D, A, or R) as noted in the preceding question. _____

Chapter 4

32. List five indications for documentation.

A._____

B._____

C._____

D._____

E._____

33. Indicate whether the following guidelines for writing nursing progress notes are true or false.

	True	False
A. You may use any color ink.	___	___
B. Do not skip lines.	___	___
C. You may use any abbreviation you want.	___	___
D. Information documented on flow sheets has to be repeated in the narrative note.	___	___
E. You may use the pronoun I.	___	___
F. Line out any unused space at the end of a note.	___	___
G. You may use ditto marks.	___	___
H. You may express opinions.	___	___
I. You should not criticize or blame other team members.	___	___
J. You may back date records.	___	___
K. You should insert forgotten information in your previous notes when you remember the information.	___	___

34. List ten types of information that must be documented.

A._____

B._____

C._____

D._____

E._____

F._____

G._____

H._____

I._____

J._____

Chapter 5

35. Name three times to document a summary of patient care.

    A._____

    B._____

    C._____

36. Write an admission note on a person admitted with asthma and no other medical problems. Use the following nursing diagnosis: impaired gas exchange, activity intolerance, and high risk for infection. (Other diagnoses would, of course, be valid, but the exercise is limited to these three.) Use your own data to write an appropriate note.

37. A properly written evaluative statement consists of what two components?

   A._____

   B._____

38. Name three times when you will write an evaluative statement.

   A._____

   B._____

   C._____

39. Define objective data._____

   _____

   _____

40. When writing an evaluation note, what two pieces of information must you convey to the reader?

A._____

B._____

41. Name three places to collect data to help write summary or evaluative statements.

A._____

B._____

C._____

42. List three effects of evaluative statements on the care plan.

A._____

B._____

C._____

43. Change the following subjective statements to objective statements.

A. Patient is anxious.

B. Voiding well.

Chapter 6

44. Write an evaluative statement based on the following information. The patient is a 45-year-old woman who has COPD. The nursing diagnosis is: gas exchange, impaired, related to altered oxygen delivery. Yesterday, she was confused all the time. Write a note reflecting improvement of her status.

45. If you cannot document immediately after an event, list three things that you can do or review to ensure that you document patient care completely.

    A._____

    B._____

    C._____

46. Write a note showing improvement in the patient's condition given the following information: The patient suffers from infectious mononucleosis; nursing diagnosis to address is fatigue related to decreased energy production.

47. Write a note recording a telephone call to a doctor for a patient who has developed a severe nose bleed. The patient was admitted laparotomy cholecystectomy.

Chapter 7

48. Name five uses of flow sheets or other forms.

   A._____

   B._____

   C._____

   D._____

   E._____

49. If you document on a form with your initials, how can someone else identify whose initials they belong to?

   _____

   _____

50. Identify two of the three major traps a nurse can fall into when documenting on a flow sheet.

   A._____

   _____

   B._____

   _____

51. True or false. When charting on flow sheets, the basic guidelines, as outlined in Chapter 4, regarding progress notes will not apply. _____

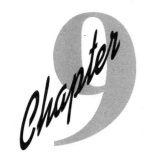

Test

Answers

The following are answers to the test questions from Chapter 8. Remember: When you were asked to write a progress note, you had to supply your own information. Therefore, your answers will vary from those shown here.

Chapter 1

1. According to the ANA's definition of nursing, nurses diagnosis and treat the *human responses* to actual or potential health problems.

2. You document to meet the needs of whom?

   A. *The patient*
   B. *The practitioner, yourself*
   C. *The agency or institution*

3. The first reason you document is to *provide high-quality care.*

4. List six reasons you document. *Communication between health team members, care provided, outcomes of care provided, patient teaching, legal, coordination of care, DRG assignment, reimbursement, continuing education, research, and Continuous Quality Improvement*

5. Why is it important to document the patient's response to the care that has been given? *So that the health care team can evaluate the effectiveness of the plan of care.*

6. True or false. You will be sued because you documented poorly. *False*

7. Patients sue nursing professionals because they have *suffered some type of emotional or physical injury*

8. True or false. Third-party payers will reimburse the hospital for any supplies as long as they are properly charged for. *False* If false what must you do to ensure proper reimbursement? *The documentation must reflect the use of the equipment and supplies.*

9. What professional organization sets standards of care for nurses? *American Nurses' Association (ANA)*

10. You are given legal permission to work as a nurse by the *Nurse Practice Act,* which is administered by the *State Board of Nursing,* and both are created under *state codes.*

11. What organization surveys a hospital to see whether the institution is meeting established standards? *Joint Commission of Accreditation of Healthcare Organizations (JCAHO)*

12. If your institution does not pass the above survey what is the impact on the institution? *Could be denied reimbursement from insurance companies, Medicare, and Medicaid.*

13. What are the standards called that are written by your institution? *Policies and procedures.*

14. True or False. Abbreviations are universal and any abbreviation may be used in any institution or agency you work in. *False*

15. What regulatory agencies mandate your documentation responsibilities? *Nurse Practice Act, ANA Standards of Care, JCAHO Standards, other regulatory agencies.*

Chapter 2

16. Your practice is defined and based on the *nursing* process.

17. List the components of the process and what occurs in each step.

   A. *Assessment: the systematic collection of data regarding the patient's health status, current problems, and ability for self-care.*
   B. *Nursing Diagnosis: the identification of those problems that the nurse can treat.*
   C. *Expected Outcomes and Care Plan: identification of goals to be achieved by the care that will be given to achieve those goals.*
   D. *Implementation: putting the care plan into action. Doing the hands on care.*
   E. *Evaluation: deciding whether or not the plan of care is effective.*

18. Name the form on which you document patient information on admission to your institution. *Nursing admission assessment*

19. On what form do you document all components of the process? *Nursing progress notes*

20. True or false. Your nursing diagnosis must indicate a need for nursing care. *True* If false, what should it indicate? *N/A*

21. After making a diagnosis, you must *validate* it with the patient. Why? *To prevent wasting time by having an improper diagnosis.*

22. Identify which component of the process is addressed in the following notes?

Explained the importance of and demonstrated the use of the incentive spirometer. *Implementation*

Abdomen soft, bowel sounds present, passing flatus. *Assessment if used in the admission note. Evaluation if noted in later progress notes.*

23. A NANDA Nursing Diagnosis can address which two types of problem? A. *Actual* B. *High-risk for*

24. The following are two NANDA Nursing Diagnoses. If they are correct as written, write "correct" in the space. If they are incorrect, rewrite them.

A. Noncompliance related to ignorance. *This is a value judgment. Correct: Noncompliance related to fear.*
B. Fear related to unfamiliarity with hospitals. *Correct*

25. Indicate which of the following guidelines for writing NANDA nursing diagnosis are incorrect.

A. Focus on a nurse's task. *Incorrect*
B. The second part of diagnosis identifies the factors that are believed to be causing or contributing to the problem. *Correct*
C. A single symptom can be used as the human response part of the diagnosis. *Incorrect*

Chapter 3

26. List four different formats of nursing documentation.

A. *Narrative*
B. *SOAP(IE)(IER)*
C. *Charting by Exception*
D. *Focus*

27. In which documentation format would you find the following type of note?

   A. D: Wound drainage light green with a foul odor, edge of wound black. Temperature 100.9°F.
A: Sterile dressing done.Old dressing 3/4 saturated with light green drainage.
                       A. *FOCUS*

   B. S: I have trouble getting my breath.
O: R 26 using accessory muscles with respiration. Crackles heard in both lower lobes. T 101.4°F.
A: Ineffective breathing patterns
P: Elevate head of bed, call Dr., push fluids, incentive spirometer q1h.
                       B. *SOAP*

28. Which documentation system sets Standards of Practice and requires the nurse to document only if the patient falls outside of the established norm? *Charting by Exception*

29. Explain what each letter of the acronym SOAP means and what type of information is documented in that section of a SOAP note.

   S: *Subjective: information that the patient provides.*
   O: *Objective: information that is collected through physical assessment, observation, monitoring, or laboratory data or information obtained from anyone other than the patient.*
   A: *Assessment: (re)statement of the nursing diagnosis and identification of progress toward the expected outcomes.*
   P: *Plans: what you plan to do now or in the future for this patient.*

30. A Focus note is divided into three parts: date/time, the focus, and the progress note. What are the three components of a Focus progress note, and what information is documented in each section?

A. *Data: information, subjective or objective, regarding the patient.*
B. *Action: anything past, present, or future that you have done or will do for the patient.*
C. *Response: how the patient responded to the medical or nursing care.*

31. True or false. Every Focus progress note must contain all three component (D, A, or R) as noted in the preceding question. *False*

Chapter 4

32. List five indications for documentation. *Admission, changes or lack of change in patient's condition, new nursing diagnosis, problems resolved, pre/post procedure, refusal of treatment, adverse reactions, patient injury, codes, telephone calls, occurrence of error or mistakes, spiritual interventions, living will declarations, unexpected events, transfers, and discharge.*

33. Indicate whether the following guidelines for writing nursing progress notes are true or false.

	True	False
A. You may use any color ink.		X
B. Do not skip lines.	X	
C. You may use any abbreviation you want.		X
D. Information documented on flow sheets has to be repeated in the narrative note.		X
E. You may use the pronoun I.	X	

	True	False
F. Line out any unused space at the end of a note.	X	
G. You may use ditto marks.		X
H. You may express opinions.		X
I. You should not criticize or blame other team members.	X	
J. You may back date records.		X
K. You should insert forgotten information in your previous notes when you remember the information.		X

34. List ten types of information that must be documented. *Since the list is too lengthy to list here, please refer to Chapter 4.*

Chapter 5

35. Name three times to document a summary of patient care.

1. *Admission*
2. *On transfer*
3. *Discharge*
4. *Periodic summaries as required by institution*

36. Write an admission note on a person admitted with asthma and no other medical problems. Use the following nursing diagnosis: impaired gas exchange, activity intolerance, and high risk for infection.

| 15 Feb. 93 2130 | Admission Assessment

Impaired gas exchange Activity intolerance High risk for infection | DATA: 21 y/o female Caucasian college student admitted to 313B, at 2045, by gurney from the Emergency Room accompanied by R. Miller, RN and N. Burns, NA and friends. Diagnosis of asthma under care of Dr. Brown, Family Practice who saw her in ED. Allergic to penicillin, develops a rash, diarrhea, and dyspnea. Developed _____(Continued) *L Martino RN* |
|---|---|---|

(Continued)

productive cough, white thick sputum, yesterday while hiking in the mountain. Did not have any medication with her, last asthma attack six years ago, but came straight to ED after hiking off the mountain. BP 124/84 T 100.5°F P 112 R 28. Inspiratory and expiratory wheeze in all lung fields. Not using accessory muscles. Color pale, skin warm and damp. Thick, white sputum produced with frequent cough. Reports being extremely tired, needs assistance moving from gurney to bed. Has only slept about 2 hours in last 36 due to cough keeping her awake last night. Mucous membranes dry and intact. Complaining of thirst. Skin turgor decreased with very little tenting. Reports BP normally 120s/80s. ACTION: Helped to bed, head of bed in high Fowler's. O_2 2 L/minute by nasal cannula. IV of D_5W @ 250cc/hr and IV aminophylline @ 35mg/hr, both IVs on pump. Humidifier @ bedside, with heavy mist directed at face. Called mother at her request and explained situation. Mother talked with friends and will be here tomorrow from out of town. All valuables previously given to friends. Refer to care plan for the specific plan of care. Side rails up, given call light. DATA: Dozing between coughing spells, which come every 10–15 minutes. Has drank 400cc of water since admission with assistance. —————————————— L Martino RN

Notes will vary. Your note should answer the following questions: Did you include the points in Chapter 4, which should be listed in an admission note. Did you address the symptoms that you would expect to see with an asthmatic patient? You will note I did not list the complete nursing diagnosis. Each facility has its own guidelines. Some will want the complete diagnosis listed when first documented; others will want the complete diagnosis only on the nursing care plan. You may want to write a discharge note on this patient.

37. A properly written evaluative statement consists of what two components?

    A. *Data on which judgment is based*
    B. *Professional judgment*

38. Name three times when you will write an evaluative statement.

    A. *After completion of admission assessment*
    B. *Reassessment of patient and plan of care*
    C. *When writing discharge assessment of each active problem*

39. Define objective data. *Measurable and verifiable information. Information is collected from physical assessment, observations, monitoring, laboratory data, or data supplied by someone other than the patient.*

40. When writing an evaluation note, what two pieces of information must you convey to the reader?

    A. *Exactly what you are evaluating*
    B. *What you are basing your evaluation on*

41. Name three places to collect data to help write summary or evaluative statements.

    A. *Laboratory data and x-ray reports*
    B. *Procedures results*
    C. *Graphic flow sheets*
    D. *Previous professional notes*
    E. *Physical reassessment*
    F. *Observations*

42. List three effects of evaluative statements on the care plan.

    A. *Further assessment and new diagnosis developed*
    B. *Continuation of the plan as written*

C. *Continuation of the plan with increased effort*
D. *Modification of the plan of care*
E. *A combination of all of the above*
F. *Resolution of the diagnosis*

43. Change the following subjective statements to objective statements.

    A. Patient is anxious.

    Patient has been pacing his room for the last hour. Muscles tight with hands balled into fist. When approached, snaps at staff with curt replies and said there is nothing to talk about.

    B. Voiding well.

    Foley out at 0930, after balloon deflated. Voided spontaneously @ 1230 & 1545 for amounts of 250cc & 325cc, respectively.

44. Write an evaluative statement based on the following information. The patient is a 45-year-old woman who has COPD. The nursing diagnosis is: gas exchange, impaired, related to altered oxygen delivery. Yesterday, she was confused all the time. Write a note reflecting improvement of her status.

Gas exchange: impaired	DATA: Awake and oriented to person all day, but could not remember place and time 50% of time when questioned. Today able to follow simple commands. Rales throughout both lungs, but amount has decreased in intensity at 1300 compared to 0800 assessment. Continues with productive cough of thick green sputum.——————— ACTION: Keep HOB @ 45°. Incentive spirometry done q2h. Encouraging fluids.——————— RESPONSE: Continues to improve compared to yesterday.———————*B. Alcorn LPN*

Chapter 6

45. If you cannot document immediately after an event, list three things that you can do or review to ensure that you document patient care completely.

    A. *Keep notes on report sheet*
    B. *Review nursing care plan*
    C. *Review doctor's orders*
    D. *Review Kardex*
    E. *Review previous nursing notes*

46. Write a note showing improvement in the patient's condition given the following information: The patient suffers from infectious mononucleosis; nursing diagnosis to address is fatigue related to decreased energy production. This note is written at 1100.

Fatigue	DATA: Setting on side of bed for breakfast this AM, first time since admission "I feel a little better today, I want to listen to the races today if possible." Slept for hour after shower, first shower since admission. Talking with roommate during breakfast.———————— ACTION: Encouraged to sleep when sleepy, not to worry that he is sleeping to much. Alternate activity with rest periods.———————— RESPONSE: Activity level increasing. Feeling stronger. *J. Hudson RN*

47. Write a note recording a telephone call to a doctor for a patient who has developed a severe nose bleed. The patient was admitted for laparotomy cholecystectomy.

Nose- bleed	DATA: Nose started to bleed @ 1415 from L nares. Started as trickle now dripping steadily, has saturated two 4x4 pads in last five minutes. Nares moist. Unable to see site of bleeding. Patient swallowing blood, able to visualize blood in back of throat. B/P 140/88 P 78. Has no history of epistaxis.———————— ACTION: Positioned patient in high Fowler's. Ice applied to nose and posterior neck. Notified Dr. Williams at 1430 of nosebleed that is not responding to nursing interventions, B/P, patient swallowing blood. Awaiting Dr.'s arrival on ward. Monitoring vital signs and bleeding, providing emotional support, J. Wallace LPN @ bedside.———————————— *L Baker RN*

(Continued) RESPONSE: Lying quietly in bed with eyes closed. Epistaxis
continues. ————————————————— *L. Baker RN*

Chapter 7

48. Name five uses of flow sheets or other forms. *I & O, activity of daily living, safety, wound monitoring, data of monitoring activities, physical assessments, patient education, admission assessments, and discharge summaries.*

49. If you document on a form with your initials, how can someone else identify whose initials they belong to? *By looking at the signature area of each form. On any form where documentation is done with initials, you must sign that area with your initials, signature, and credentials.*

50. Identify two of the three major traps a nurse can fall into when documenting on a flow sheet.

    A. *Not looking at what your are documenting.*
    B. *Underrating the importance of the documentation done on a flow sheet to the patient's care and to meeting legal protection needs.*
    C. *Depending too much on flow sheets to cover your documentation responsibilities.*

51. True or false. When charting on flow sheets, the basic guidelines, outlined in Chapter 4, regarding progress notes will not apply. *False*

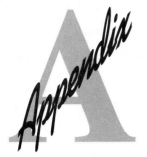

List of NANDA Nursing Diagnoses*

Exchanging

Altered Nutrition: More than body requirements
Altered Nutrition: Less than body requirements
Altered Nutrition: Potential for more than body requirement
High Risk for Infection
High Risk for Altered Body Temperature
Hypothermia
Hyperthermia
Ineffective Thermoregulation
Dysreflexia
Constipation†
Perceived Constipation
Colonic Constipation
Diarrhea†
Bowel Incontinence†
Altered Urinary Elimination
Stress Incontinence
Reflex Incontinence
Urge Incontinence
Functional Incontinence
Total Incontinence
Urinary Retention
Altered (Specify Type) Tissue Perfusion (renal, cerebral, cardiopulmonary, gastrointestinal, peripheral)†

Fluid Volume Excess
Fluid Volume Deficit
High Risk for Fluid Volume Deficit
Decreased Cardiac Output†
Impaired Gas Exchange
Ineffective Airway Clearance
Ineffective Breathing Pattern
Inability to Sustain Spontaneous Ventilation‡
Dysfunctional Ventilatory Weaning Response (DVWR)‡
High Risk for Injury
High Risk for Suffocation
High Risk for Poisoning
High Risk for Trauma
High Risk for Aspiration
High Risk for Disuse Syndrome
Altered Protection
Impaired Tissue Integrity
Altered Oral Mucous Membrane†
Impaired Skin Integrity
High Risk for Impaired Skin Integrity

‡ New diagnostic categories approved 1992
† Categories with modified label terminology

* Reprinted with permission from North American Nursing Diagnosis Association (1992). NANDA Nursing Diagnosis: Definitions and Classifications 1992–1993, © Philadelphia: NANDA, pages 6–9.

Communicating
Impaired Verbal Communication
Relating

Relating
Impaired Social Interaction
Social Isolation
Altered Role Performance†
Altered Parenting
High Risk for Altered Parenting
Sexual Dysfunction
Altered Family Processes
Caregiver Role Strain‡
High Risk for Caregiver Role Strain‡
Parental Role Conflict
Altered Sexuality Patterns

Valuing
Spiritual Distress (distress of the human
spirit)

Choosing
Ineffective Individual Coping
Impaired Adjustment
Defensive Coping
Ineffective Denial
Ineffective Family Coping: Disabling
Ineffective Family Coping: Compromised
Family Coping: Potential for Growth
Ineffective Management of Therapeutic
Regimen (Individuals)‡
Noncompliance (Specify)
Decisional Conflict (Specify)
Health-Seeking Behaviors (Specify)

Moving
Impaired Physical Mobility
High Risk for Peripheral Neurovascular
Dysfunction‡
Activity Intolerance
Fatigue
High Risk for Activity Intolerance
Sleep Pattern Disturbance
Diversional Activity Deficit
Impaired Home Maintenance Management
Altered Health Maintenance
Feeding Self-Care Deficit†
Impaired Swallowing
Ineffective Breast-feeding

Interrupted Breast-feeding‡
Effective Breast-feeding
Ineffective Infant Feeding Pattern‡
Bathing/Hygiene Self-Care Deficit†
Dressing/Grooming Self-Care Deficit†
Toileting Self-Care Deficit†
Altered Growth and Development
Relocation Stress Syndrome‡

Perceiving
Body Image Disturbance‡
Self-Esteem Disturbance‡
Chronic Low Self Esteem
Situational Low Self Esteem
Personal Identity Disturbance‡
Sensory/Perceptual Alterations (Specify)
(Visual, auditory, kinesthetic,
gustatory, tactile, olfactory)
Unilateral Neglect
Hopelessness
Powerlessness

Knowing
Knowledge Deficit (Specify)
Altered Thought Processes

Feeling
Pain†
Chronic Pain
Dysfunctional Grieving
Anticipatory Grieving
High Risk for Violence: Self-directed or
directed at others
High Risk for Self-Mutilation‡
Post-Trauma Response
Rape-Trauma Syndrome
Rape-Trauma Syndrome: Compound Reaction
Rape-Trauma Syndrome: Silent Reaction
Anxiety
Fear

Bibliography

Adams, C. (1989). Computer-Generated Medication Administration Records. *Nursing Management, 20*(7), 22–23.

American Nurses Association. (1980). *Nursing: A Social Policy Statement.* Washington: Author.

American Nurses Association. (1991). *Standards of Clinical Nursing Practice.* Washington: Author.

Boulder Community Hospital. (1992). *Ob/Gyn Assessment Flow Sheet.* Boulder, CO: Unpublished form.

Brider, P. (1991). Who Killed the Nursing Care Plan? *American Journal of Nursing, 93*(5), 35–39.

Burke, L. J., & Murphy, J. (1988). *Charting By Exception.* Media, PA: Harwal Publishing Company.

Butler, P. (1991). The Nursing Shortage: The Legal Impact on Documentation. *The Journal of Continuing Education in Nursing, 22*(5), 189–191.

Caine, R. M., & Bufalino, P. M. (1991). *Nursing Care Planning Guides for Adults* (2nd ed.). Baltimore: Williams & Wilkins.

Carpenito, L. J. (1991). *Handbook of Nursing Diagnosis.* Philadelphia: J. B. Lippincott Company.

Carpenito, L. J. (1991). Has JCAHO eliminated care plans? *American Nurse, 23*(6), 6.

Cline, A. (1989). Streamlined Documentation Through Exceptional Charting. *Nursing Management, 20*(2), 62–64.

Coles, M. C., & Fullenwider, S. D. (1988). Documentation: Managing the Dilemma. *Nursing Management, 19*(12), 65–66, 70, 72.

Courmoyer, C. P. (1989). *The Nurse Manager and the Law.* Rockville, MD: Aspen Publisher.

Cushing, M. (1992). *Nursing Jurisprudence.* Rockville, MD: Aspen Publisher.

Decker, P. J., & Sullivan, E. J. (1992). *Nursing Administration: A Micro/Macro Approach for Effective Nurse Executives.* Norwalk, CT: Appleton & Lange.

DiBlasi, M. (1992). Revitalizing a Documentation System. *Rehabilitation Nursing, 17*(1), 27–29.

Dill-Calloway, S. (1991). *Ohio Nursing Law.* Cleveland: Banks Baldwin Law Publishing.

Dill-Calloway, S. (1993). *The Law for Nurses Who Supervise and Manage Others.* Eau Claire, WI: Professional Education Systems.

Doenges, M. E., & Moorhouse, M. F. (1991). *Nursing Diagnoses with Interventions.* (3rd ed.). Philadelphia: F. A. Davis Company.

Edelstein, J. (1990). Study of Nursing Documentation. *Nursing Management, 21*(11), 40–43, 46.

Eggland, E. T. (1988). Charting How and Why to Document Your Care Daily—and Fully. *Nursing88, 18*(11), 76–79, 81–84.

Feutz-Harter, S. (1989). Legal Insights. *Journal of Nursing Administration, 19*(12), 7–9.

Feutz-Harter, S. (1991). *Nursing and the Law.* Eau Claire, WI: Professional Education Systems.

Fischbach, F. T. (1991). *Documenting Care Communication, the Nursing Process and Documentation Standards.* Philadelphia: F. A. Davis Co.

Fox-Ungar, E., Newell, G., & Guilbault, K. (1989). Documentation: Communicating Professionalism. *Nursing Management, 20*(1), 65–66, 68, 70.

Georgia Board of Nursing. (1990). *Georgia Registered Professional Nurse Practice Act.* Charlottesville, VA: The Michie Company.

Georgia Board of Practical Nursing. (1989). *Georgia Practical Nurse Practice Act.* Charlottesville, VA: The Michie Company.

Glanze, W. D. (Ed.). (1990). *Mosby's Medical, Nursing, and Allied Health Dictionary.* St. Louis: Mosby-Year Book.

Goldstein, A. S., Perdew, S., & Pruitt, S. (1989). *The Nurse's Legal Advisor.* Philadelphia: J. B. Lippincott.

Gove, P. B. (Ed.). (1986). *Webster's Third New International Dictionary.* Springfield, MA: Merriam-Webster Inc.

Greve, P. (1991). Advance Directives—What The New Law Means For You. *RN, 54*(11), 63–64, 66.

Guido, G. W. (1988). *Legal Issues in Nursing.* Norwalk, CT: Appleton & Lange.

Hirshfield-Bartek, J., Dow, K. H., & Creaton, E. (1990). Decreasing Documentation Time Using a Patient Self-Assessment Tool. *Oncology Nursing Forum, 17,* 251–255.

Kabl, K., Ivancin, L., & Fubrmann, M. (1991). Automated Nursing Documentation System Provides a Favorable Return on Investment. *Journal of Nursing Administration, 21*(11), 44–51.

Kleiber, C., & Chase, L. (1989). Solving Documentation Problems With a Pediatric Flow Sheet. *Pediatric Nursing, 15,* 253–256, 267.

Knapp-Spooner, C., & Brett, J. (1992). Less Is More: A Med/Surg Flow Sheet. *RN, 55*(3), 36–39.

Knights, S. (1989). Assessment To Discharge, This Form Does It All. *RN, 52*(7), 36–40.

Ignatavicius, D. D., & Bayne, M. V. (1991). *Medical-Surgical Nursing A Nursing Process Approach.* Philadelphia: W. B. Saunders Company.

Iyer, P. (1991). New Trends in Charting. *Nursing91, 21*(1), 48–50.

Iyer, P. (1991). Thirteen Charting Rules. *Nursing91, 21*(6), 40–44, 47.

Iyer, P. (1991) Six More Charting Rules. *Nursing91, 21*(7), 34–39.

Iyer, P., Taptich, B. J., & Bernocchi-Losey, D. (1991). *Nursing Process and Nursing Diagnosis.* Philadelphia: W. B. Saunders Company.

Joint Commission on Accreditation of Healthcare Organizations. (1993). *Accreditation Manual for Hospitals, Volume 1 Standards.* Oakbrook Terrance, IL: Author.

Lampe, S. S. (1985). Focus Charting: Streamlining Documentation. *Nursing Management. 16*((7), 43–44, 46.

Lampe, S. S. (1988). *Focus Charting™.* Minneapolis: Creative Nursing Management, Inc.

Lang, N. M., & Gebbie, K. (1988). Nursing Taxonomy: NANDA and ANA Joint Venture toward ICD-10CM. In R. Carroll-Johnson (Ed.). *Classification of Nursing Diagnosis, Proceeding of the Eighth Conference.* (pp. 11–17). Philadelphia: J. B. Lippincott Company.

Loeb, S. (Ed.). (1991). *Illustrated Manual of Nursing Practice.* Springhouse, PA: Springhouse Corporation.

Loeb, S. (Ed.). (1992). *Law & Ethics.* Springhouse, PA: Springhouse Corporation.

Loeb, S. (Ed.). (1992). *Better Documentation.* Springhouse, PA: Springhouse Corporation.

Lucatorto, M., Petras, D., Drew, L., & Zbuckvich, I. (1991). Documentation A Focus for Cost Savings. *Journal of Nursing Administration,* 21(3), 32–36.

Marrelli, T. M. (1992). *Nursing Documentation Handbook*. St. Louis: Mosby Year Book.

Montemuro, M. (1988). CORE Documentation: A Complete System for Charting Nursing Care. *Nursing Management*, *19*(18), 28–32.

Moorhouse, M. F., & Doenges, M. E. (1990). *Nurse's Clinical Pocket Manual: Nursing Diagnoses, Care Planning, and Documentation*. Philadelphia: F. A. Davis Company.

Murphy, J., & Burke, L. J. (1990). Charting by Exception. *Nursing90*, *20*(5), 65, 68–69.

Neubauer, M. P. (1990). Careful Charting—Your Best Defense. *RN*, *53*((11), 77–80.

North American Nursing Diagnosis Association (1992). *NANDA Nursing Diagnosis: Definitions and Classification 1992-1993*. Philadelphia: Author.

Parsek, J. D. (1991). Did JCAHO Abolish Care Plans! Yes! *American Nurse*, *23*(8), 6.

Potter, P. A., & Perry, A. G. (1989). *Fundamentals of Nursing*. St. Louis: Mosby Year Book.

Reiley, P. J., & Stengrevics, S. S. (1989). Change-of-Shift Report: Put it in Writing! *Nursing Management*, *20*(9), 54–56.

Schmidt, D., Gathers, B., Stewart, M., Tyler, C., Hawkins, M., & Denton, K.(1990). Charting for Accountability. *Nursing Management*, 21(11), 50–52.

Thompson, J. M., McFarland, G. K., Hirsch, J. E., Tucker, S. M., & Bowers, A. C. (1989). *Mosby's Manual of Clinical Nursing* (2nd ed.). St. Louis: Mosby Year Book.

Warne, M. A., & McWeeny, M. C. (1991). Managing the Cost of Documentation: The FACT Charting System. *Nursing Economics*, *9*, 181–187.

Wayne Memorial Hospital. (1991). *Nursing Admission Assessment*. Jesup, GA: Unpublished form.

Index

S

Special practice groups 13, 19
Spiritual interventions 62, 112
Standards
   ANA's: of care 14
   JCAHO's: nursing 17, 18
   nursing 45
   practice 13
State and federal government 18
State Boards of Nursing 13, 14
   responsibilities 15
Subjective information 42, 91
   definition of 42
Subjective statements 91, 92
Summary notes 77
   admission 78
   death 88
   discharge 85
   transfer 83
   types 78

T

Techniques of documentation 65
Telephone calls 60, 108
Transfer 63, 83
   type of information 63

U

Unexpected events 63
Unscheduled medications 61, 111

Order Form

To order copies of this book, send check or money order and coupon to:
Awareness Productions
P.O. Box 85
Tipp City, Ohio 45371-0085

Make check or money order payable to **Awareness Productions**. Copies of this coupon or letters are accepted .

Return policy: Refunds will be given on all returned unmarked books.

Complete the following. Print clearly or type.

Title	Qty	Price	Total
Documentation Skills for Quality Patient Care		$18.95	
Shipping: 1 Book = $1.75 Each additional book = $1.00 each	Total		
	6% Tax (Ohio only)		
	Shipping		
	Total		

For large orders, contact Awareness Productions or the medical book distributor: J. A. Majors Company, 1851 Diplomat, P.O. Box 819074, Dallas, TX 75381-9074.

Name: _____

Address: _____

_____

_____

_____

Expect delivery in four to six weeks.